2019

SEPTEMBER–DECEMBER

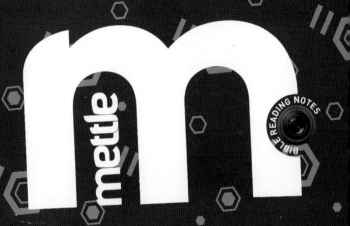

mettle

BIBLE READING NOTES

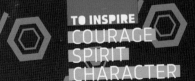

TO INSPIRE
COURAGE
SPIRIT
CHARACTER

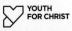

YOUTH FOR CHRIST

CWR

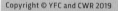

CONTENTS

Welcome to

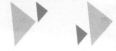

mettle

COURAGE SPIRIT CHARACTER...

Many people own a Bible or have one on their phones, but what's it all about? Our core readings unpack the story of the Bible and what it means for us today. We've also got three great topics to explore: family, celebrate and integrity. Sometimes family life is fun; sometimes it's a nightmare! Let's see what the Bible says about getting on with others and celebrating good times. Finally, we will be thinking about integrity and how to live in line with what we believe.

In this issue, readers have shared their thoughts about the Bible in a new 'Share' feature. If you would like to share something about God, your faith, or how the Bible helps you, send an email to mettle@cwr.org.uk

We would love to hear from you!

The *Mettle* Team

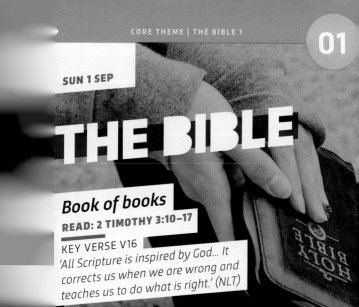

SUN 1 SEP

THE BIBLE

Book of books

READ: 2 TIMOTHY 3:10–17

KEY VERSE V16
'All Scripture is inspired by God... It corrects us when we are wrong and teaches us to do what is right.' (NLT)

The Bible remains the world's bestseller year after year. Many people around the world own or have access to a Bible. But have you actually read it? What is the Bible all about anyway?

The word 'Bible' is derived from the Greek word meaning 'books'. That's a big clue because the Bible is a mini library of writings, which are divided into Testaments – Old and New. The Old Testament contains all the books written before the birth of Jesus, and the New Testament all those books written after Jesus was born.

Some of the books originate from ancient cultures and so they may seem bizarre with lists of names, weird rules and strange customs. That doesn't mean they are irrelevant now, but just need to be interpreted. Today's passage says that the Bible is inspired by God to help us know how to live and relate to others. When we understand the big picture of the Bible, we realise that this big, old book speaks to us in new and exciting ways.

The Bible also tells us a story. A story that spans thousands of years, and consists of many characters, dramas and miracles. It's God's story of how He loves us and wants us to love Him too. We're going to be discovering this story in three sections on the Bible.

With so many different books (66 in total!), you might wonder where on earth to start. It's like scrolling through shows on Netflix and not knowing what to watch first. Starting to watch a show at season six when there are 30 seasons would be a bit confusing. We're going to start at season one – Genesis.

Pray

Holy Spirit, as I read the Bible, please open my heart and mind to understand Your amazing plan for the world and for me. Amen.

And so it begins

READ: GENESIS 2:4–9,15–17,19–25

KEY VERSE V7
'Then the LORD God formed a man from the dust of the ground and breathed into his nostrils the breath of life, and the man became a living being.'

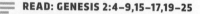

Have you ever viewed the world using Google Earth? It's amazing how we can see the whole planet on our screens and then zoom in on a continent, a country, a county, a town and even a street. Genesis chapter 1 zooms out to give us a speedy overview to the creation of the world. Light and darkness, land and water, trees and plants, sun and moon, bird and sea creatures were created with very little detail. In Genesis chapter 2, however, the creation process slows down and zooms in on God's masterpiece: men and women. Humans were, and still are, the best example of God's creativity.

Adam and Eve were not created just so that God would have someone to talk to; they had a particular job to do. God wanted to give His proudest achievement the privilege of looking after Earth. That is still God's goal for us today: to work in ways that benefit the whole world. We can all do things such as helping our neighbour, looking after our pets, taking care of a garden or doing some voluntary work. This kind of 'work' is helpful to others but is beneficial to us too. Instead of thinking of work as a chore, we can be energised and fulfilled when we do something for God. What 'work' could you do for God?

CORE THEME | THE BIBLE 1

66 *Share*

'I think that the Bible is helpful and interesting. I sometimes read it with my friends on FaceTime.' (Josh, 16)

Shadow of a doubt

READ: GENESIS 3:1–19

KEY VERSE V11
*'Have you eaten from the tree from which
I commanded you not to eat?'*

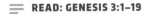

It was all going so well. Adam and Eve were enjoying the beautiful Garden of Eden. All they had to do was follow one simple rule: don't eat the fruit of the tree in the middle of the garden. Sounds easy, and at first the couple were happy to comply. That was until Satan, in the form of a crafty snake, sowed seeds of doubt in their minds. Why has God commanded that? Doesn't He want the best for you?

These doubts coupled with the fact that the fruit looked so darn good, quickly persuaded Eve to grab some and taste it. Big mistake! They had chosen to disobey God and now they had to face the consequences. The good times were over and they had to leave Eden.

Adam and Even had been created to enjoy a special closeness with God but they had spoilt it by listening to and believing the lies of Satan, rather than God. What God wanted with Adam and Eve is the same thing that He wants with us: a close relationship. In the Bible, we will see that, time and time again, God seeks to restore that broken friendship. Some things in the Bible are difficult for us to grasp but there is one consistent theme: God loves us and He wants the best for us.

❝ *Share*

'My favourite Bible verse is Lamentations 3:22–23: "Because of the Lᴏʀᴅ's great love we are not consumed, for his compassions never fail. They are new every morning; great is your faithfulness"' (Ethan, 17)

Strange long-term plan

READ: GENESIS 11:27–32; 12:1–9

KEY VERSES 12:2–3
*'I will make you into a great nation, and I will bless you…
and all peoples on earth will be blessed through you.'*

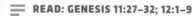

'If at first you don't succeed, try, try again.' This was clearly God's personal motto. Garden of Eden, Noah and the Flood, the Tower of Babel are all stories about people not listening to God. In all three examples, God responds to disobedience with judgment, but He doesn't give up on His people.

Abram is pivotal to God's two-part plan to restore our perfect relationship with Him, if we want it. Part one – God would make Abram the leader of a great nation, give that nation a land and bless the people. Part two – God would use this nation to be a blessing to the whole world. Many years later, a descendant of Abram, Jesus Christ, would enable all people to know a close relationship with God.

This sounds great apart from the fact that Abram is very old, doesn't have any children and lives miles away from God's intended Promised Land in Canaan. So how is God's restoration plan going to pan out? Who knew? But Abram took God at His word and set off towards Canaan. Abram had faith and confidence in God. Today, as we read and trust God's Word and put our confidence in His Son, Jesus Christ, we are included in the blessing that was promised to Abram. When God was addressing Abram, He had you and me in mind.

CORE THEME | THE BIBLE 1

 Share

'My favourite Bible character is Samson because he was a good role model of someone who followed God's Word.' (Cam, 15)

Hand of God

READ: EXODUS 13:3–21

KEY VERSE V3
'Then Moses said to the people, "Commemorate this day, the day you came out of Egypt, out of the land of slavery."'

Brexit. Like it or loath it, this word sums up the process of Britain exiting the European Union. The word 'exit' originates from Latin whereas the word 'exodus' originates from Greek. Both words mean 'the way out'.

The book of Exodus began with God's promise to Abram that he would be the father of a great nation with a land of their own looking like it has hit the rocks. A great famine in Canaan has forced Abram's grandson, Jacob, and his family to travel to Egypt for food where they remained for around 400 years. During that time, the Israelites (Abram's descendants) grew in number and began to pose a threat to Pharaoh, the Egyptian leader. As a precaution, Pharaoh forces them to become slaves and gives the order for all male babies to be killed at birth.

Things looked bad for the Israelites, but God had not forgotten His promise and had a plan that was called 'Moses'. God was working behind the scenes from the moment Moses was born to ensure that he would be the best person to confront Pharaoh and tell him to let God's people go. After some pretty miraculous signs of God's power, the Israelites were finally allowed to leave Egypt – it was a day definitely worth remembering and celebrating!

 Share

'The Bible has helped me to know what to say in certain situations.' (Daniel, 15)

CORE THEME | THE BIBLE 1

Team rules

READ: EXODUS 20:1–21

KEY VERSE V6
'I lavish unfailing love... on those who love me and obey my commands.' (NLT)

'Free at last, free at last! Thank God Almighty, we are free at last.' These words said by Martin Luther King Jr in 1963 would have been sentiments felt by the Israelites as they left Egypt and embraced their new life of freedom.

God has rescued His people and now they are free. They gather at Mount Sinai in the desert to meet their rescuer God who asks them whether, as rescued people, they are willing to be a model community to surrounding nations who were still slaves to idolatry. To live in that freedom, they would need to follow rules and guidelines. *Wait, what? Rules to live in freedom?* Absolutely, though this seems like a paradox, God gives the Ten Commandments as a 'How to live in freedom' guide; life is much easier if everyone is on the same page. The Israelites were given freedom and now God wanted to know if they would be His representatives by following his lovingly thought-out rules.

Just as God blessed Abraham (previously called Abram) and told him that he would be a blessing to all nations, we are blessed to know the good news about Jesus and can accept the task to pass on that blessing.

Are you willing to be God's representative?

❝ *Share*

'My favourite Bible character is Jonah because he keeps his faith even when going through bizarre events.' (Marcus, 18)

CORE THEME | THE BIBLE 1

Weekend

7/8 SEP

An example to others
READ: JOSHUA 1:1–18

KEY VERSE V8
'Keep this Book of the Law always on your lips; meditate on it day and night, so that you may be careful to do everything written in it.'

Just to recap: God gave Abraham the Promised Land of Canaan; famine means that Jacob and sons leave Canaan to live in Egypt; after 400 years, they leave Egypt to go back to Canaan.

We pick up the story with the death of Moses, and Joshua being tasked with leading the people of Israel back to Canaan. The only problem now is that Canaan is inhabited by various people who will not be best pleased to have to vacate the area, so this will require going into battle. Joshua has been promised that wherever he puts his foot, God will give the Israelites the land. All he has to do is keep his heart close to God by obeying the Law of God given to Moses.

Even though Joshua is told not to be afraid as God will be with him and give him victory in battle, you might wonder why God didn't just lead His people somewhere else? Well, this might make uncomfortable reading but the sins of the people in Canaan were so horrendous that they needed to be removed permanently. God wanted to protect His people from any bad influences, and a victory over their enemies would reinforce the understanding that God was in charge.

These 'horrible biblical histories' were not God's ideal. After all, He wanted the Israelites to be a blessing to other nations. But it seems that the people in Canaan had run out of chances. Whatever the reason, Jesus' life and death shows us how to be a people of tolerance, grace, forgiveness and peace. Just as Joshua is given the land he sets foot on, we too are called to be an influence for good wherever we are and wherever we go.

Think
Where will your feet take you this week? Where could you be an influence for good?

Not licensed to build

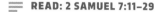

READ: 2 SAMUEL 7:11–29

KEY VERSE V22
'How great you are, Sovereign LORD! There is no one like you, and there is no God but you, as we have heard with our own ears.'

James Bond is famed for his heroic deeds, his devotion to his country and his good looks. While most people might admire 007, no one can deny that he has killed a lot of people and used a lot of women.

King David was Israel's second king and he proved to be a good choice. He had slain Goliath, been successful in battle, loved His nation and obeyed His God. Once the land of Israel seemed relatively safe and secure, David turned his attention to building a proper temple for God. But God didn't need a temple right now and even if He did, David was not the person for the job. He had fought in wars, slept with another man's wife, lied about it and then had the husband murdered. King David building a temple would be like James Bond building St. Paul's Cathedral – it just wouldn't be right.

God had a better idea. Instead of David doing something for God, God would do something for David. He was going to establish a dynasty starting with David's family. This promise was fulfilled with Jesus, David's descendant, whose kingdom is everlasting and includes *all* who truly trust Him. God's goodness to us is much greater and bigger than we can imagine.

> ## *Share*
> *'My favourite Bible verse is John 3:16 because it sums up why we believe in God.' (Daniel, 15)*

Head or heart person?

READ: PSALM 1; PSALM 23

KEY VERSE 23:6
'Surely your goodness and love will follow me all the days of my life, and I will dwell in the house of the LORD forever.'

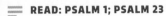

Are you an Elinor or a Marianne? If you are familiar with Jane Austen's *Sense and Sensibility*, then you will know that Elinor was the sensible and reserved sister who was always careful to do the right thing. Marianne, however, was very romantic and eager to express her emotions.

King David was actually a mix of these two personalities. He knew and followed the Law of God carefully; he even copied out the Law with his own hand. However, David was also happy to worship God through poetry, song and dancing. Many of the psalms were written by David and have inspired hymns and worship songs, that you might be familiar with.

Psalm 23 is one of the most famous passages from the Bible. It is a revealing glimpse into David's personal relationship with God. He refers to God as a shepherd who 'leads', 'refreshes', and 'guides'.

The passion expressed in the psalms reminds us that we are not just to follow God's rules but to be people who genuinely love the Lord with all our heart, soul and strength. Jesus was drawn to people who were true worshippers rather than people who were sticklers to the rules. Once we focus on being true worshippers, following God's rules will seem second-nature.

CORE THEME | THE BIBLE 1

66 *Share*

'The Bible has helped me to explore more about God, and gives me reassurance that I am loved by Him.' (Harriet, 16)

Wisdom for the road ahead

READ: PROVERBS 3:1–20

KEY VERSE V7
'Do not be wise in your own eyes; fear the LORD and shun evil.'

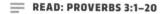

'Do. Or do not. There is no try.' This is one of Yoda's most memorable quotes from *The Empire Strikes Back**. He was the go-to source of wisdom for all would-be Jedis.

The book of Proverbs is another (maybe better?) source of wisdom that has helped followers of God when faced with life's challenges. They are not laws but helpful sayings about how life usually pans out when lived a certain way. It reminds us that God wants to help us with all aspect of our lives.

The majority of the proverbs are attributed to King Solomon who asked God for wisdom rather than riches early on in his reign (2 Chron. 1:1–12). People from all over the world came to hear the wisdom of Solomon, but being wise didn't stop him from making lots of mistakes. He had a weakness for women that led him away from God and he forced people to work on his big building projects.

In verse 7, we are reminded that while we think that we have good ideas and can figure life out, the person who puts their trust in God and obeys Him is the wisest person of all. When we ask the Holy Spirit to guide us, we can receive divine wisdom for dealing with life's issues. In what way do you need wisdom today?

> ❝ **Share**
>
> 'My favourite Bible character is Samuel because he listened when God spoke to him.' (Samuel, 16)

*20th Century Fox, 1980

Blogging

READ: ECCLESIASTES 3:1–8; 12:9–14

KEY VERSE 12:13
'Now all has been heard; here is the conclusion of the matter: Fear God and keep his commandments, for this is the duty of all mankind.'

Who's your favourite blogger or vlogger? Some of them record every aspect of their lives from what they had for breakfast to their mental health.

Eccelesiastes is believed to have been written by Solomon, a bit like an ancient form of blogging or journalling. He reflects on his own life, his successes and failures, what he has observed and his conclusions. Solomon also writes about the futility of trusting in wisdom, riches, power, and sex to bring meaning to life.

Today's reading gives us a glimpse into the inner workings of Solomon's mind and might encourage us to think about how we see the world. There is nothing wrong with stepping back and questioning things – it might even strengthen our faith.

Solomon eventually comes to the conclusion that lots of things are temporary or fleeting but the important thing to hold dear is to 'Fear God and keep his commandments'.

Why not jot down a few of your thoughts or questions about life? You could come back to them at a later date and see if you have reached any conclusions.

66 *Share*

'The Bible has helped me to become stronger in my faith, and more able to establish my own foundations and convictions in what I believe.' (Grace, 18)

CORE THEME | THE BIBLE 1

Beautifully flawed

READ: 2 KINGS 24:1–20

KEY VERSE V20
'It was because of the LORD's anger that all this happened to Jerusalem and Judah, and in the end he thrust them from his presence.'

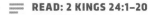

Kintsugi is the Japanese art of repairing broken pottery with gold lacquer. Rather than hiding the cracks, this method emphasises them, resulting in a beautiful piece of ceramic that reveals some of its history.

Today's reading is pretty bleak. After King Solomon (David's son) died, the kingdom of Israel spilt into two: the northern kingdom (Israel) and the southern kingdom (Judah). The people of Israel ignored repeated calls from prophets to turn back to God, until, in 722 BC, they were conquered by the Assyrians and displaced around the Assyrian empire.

Things were not looking good in Judah either. Several kings in succession 'did evil in the eyes of the LORD' (v9). Finally, the Babylonian army invaded and took all the skilled people back to Babylon. At least those deported were allowed to stay together. They soon realised that they had done wrong and began to revive their faith.

Even followers of Jesus will know bleak times. God does not promise an easy life or to protect us from the consequences of unwise choices but He promises to be with us in the pain. Sometimes, He can turn our broken times around so that, in time, they can be used to reflect God's faithfulness and everlasting love.

CORE THEME | THE BIBLE 1

💬 Share

'My favourite Bible verse is 1 Corinthians 13:4, "Love is patient, love is kind. It does not envy, it does not boast, it is not proud."' (Josh, 16)

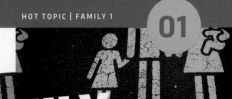

01

FAMILY

We are family

READ: GENESIS 2:18–24

KEY VERSE V18
'The LORD God said, "It is not good for the man to be alone."'

We might not choose our relatives – we might not even like them at times – but they can still enrich our lives in a very profound way.

Family is God's idea, and comes in all shapes and sizes – it's so much more than the people we're related to. There are biological families, adopted families, step-families, foster families, church families... God knows that trying to make our way through life on our own is not good for us. We're created to be in relationships with other people. Being part of a family is the best way for us to be loved, supported, encouraged, protected and guided.

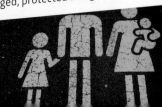

So when God made Adam, the very first human being, He made him a wonderful counterpart, Eve, so that they could be together and start a family of their own.

When a family works well, it's a wonderful thing. Hopefully, you can think of times when your family has made you feel loved, secure and hopeful. Of course, things don't always work like that. Our families can let us down too, and perhaps you can think of occasions when that has happened to you. But even when things go wrong, God still loves our families and can bless them.

In this series of readings, we'll look at all aspects of family life – the good and the bad. We'll start by looking at what's great about families, then go on to tackle how we should respond when things go wrong at home. We'll reflect on God's commands to love and forgive the people around us and discuss how that should affect our family life.

Think

What does 'family' mean to you? How do you think God wants you to relate to your family? Do you have any questions for Him about this? Write down those questions and see if He answers them over the next few weeks.

Rooted in love

☰ **READ: EPHESIANS 3:14–19**

KEY VERSES VV14–15
'I kneel before the Father, from whom every family
in heaven and on earth derives its name.'

God Himself is relational – He is one being, but at the
same time He is Father, Son and Holy Spirit, in constant
relationship with Himself. It can be a bit of a head-melt
trying to grasp the concept of the Trinity, but loving
relationships are at the core of who God is. And God didn't
create humankind because He was lonely – He made us
out of an excess of love, not a lack of community.

Today's reading from Ephesians tells us that 'every
family in heaven and on earth derives its name' from
Father God (v15). When you look at your family members,
you might think they are quite ordinary or unremarkable
– perhaps they are annoying, or maybe they're your best
friends as well as your relatives! But a family can point
towards a loving, relational God, and the more we play our
part in loving and supporting our families, the more we
can emulate the family model demonstrated by God.

Paul's letter to the Ephesians also brings us all together
as Christians in the family of Christ – the head of our
church family is God. When we remind ourselves that it's
His name that makes us a family in the first place, it ought
to be a lot easier for us to put our differences aside.

⬆ *Pray*
*This week, ask God to help you see your family as He does.
Pray for each member and ask God to make you and your
whole family a better reflection of Him.*

Honouring our parents

READ: EPHESIANS 6:1–4

KEY VERSE V1
'obey your parents in the Lord, for this is right.'

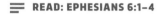

A common question people might ask after reading today's verses is this: 'What happens when my parents are wrong?' Even if you have amazing parents who do everything in your best interest, they're human beings – they won't be perfect. So are we supposed to just blindly obey whatever they ask of us, even if we think it's wrong, dangerous, or not in line with what God asks of us?

The NIV translation of the Bible puts today's verses like this: 'obey your parents *in the Lord*' (emphasis added) – in other words, within the will of God. What God thinks should be number one in our lives, and He likes us to use our common sense. But that's not a valid excuse for not taking the bins out!

Parenting is hard work, and so we can honour the parents or carers in our lives by responding positively to what they ask of us. Our habit should be to obey them and exceptions to this rule should be rare.* Let's not get distracted by judging our parents on how good a job they're doing. Instead, let's concentrate on the command that applies to us.

HOT TOPIC | FAMILY 1

🕱 *Think*

How good are you at obeying your mum and/or dad (or carer)? When you go against them, how good are your reasons? Be honest with yourself!

*If someone in your family is hurting you or abusing you, talk to an adult you trust or contact ChildLine on 0800 1111 (UK).

Disagreeing well

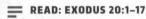

READ: EXODUS 20:1–17

KEY VERSE V12
'Honour your father and mother, so that you may live long in the land the LORD your God is giving you.'

Yesterday we mentioned how important it is to obey our parents. But the older we get, the more we realise that life isn't always that simple. What happens when we've grown up and moved out – do we still need to do everything our parents tell us to?

Of course not. It is totally possible to disagree with our parents and still honour them. For example – imagine you are applying to university. You want to study music, because it's what you're passionate about. Your parents, on the other hand, want you to study a subject that might make it 'easier' for you to get a job after graduation. Clearly, your parents are concerned for your future, and want you to have more security, more options. Our parents won't always make the right call. When we disagree with them, we can pray about it, calmly talk it over with them and show them that we still love them and respect them.

Many of us know that honouring your father and mother is one of the Ten Commandments. But did you realise that it comes with a promise? God knows that honouring our parents will bring blessings. We might not always agree with our parents, but we can always choose to honour them.

Challenge

The next time you disagree with your mum or dad, don't lose the plot. Pray about it, talk it over and ask for God's wisdom for the way forward.

HOT TOPIC | FAMILY 1

God's priorities

READ: PSALM 68:3–6

KEY VERSE V5
'Father to the fatherless, defender of widows—this is God' (NLT)

When someone in your family dies, it can be incredibly painful – especially if it's someone you were particularly close to. Perhaps you never knew one or both of your parents, and have grown up missing them. Maybe one of your siblings has moved out or gone to university, and you miss them terribly. Whatever our family situation, there will be times when we feel lonely, hurt and confused. It can be so hard to cope with change or feelings of loss. But, even in the painful times, God is still with us.

Today's key verse says a lot about who God is, and what His priorities are. He is our perfect Father, He is the one who protects the vulnerable, and He is the one who puts people around us who will help us. In the family of God, no one needs to be lonely. God cares a great deal about the 'fatherless', 'widows' and 'the lonely', so we should too. If you fall into one of those categories, spend some time talking with God and ask Him to reveal His heart for you. If not, ask Him who you could be a real friend to, and think about how you could show God's love to someone else who feels alone.

HOT TOPIC | FAMILY 1

⬆ *Pray*

If your family is going through a hard time, ask God to show you that He is with you as your perfect Father. If your family is doing OK, pray for someone you know who is going through a difficult situation with their family.

Reconcilers

READ: LUKE 1:5–25

KEY VERSE V17
'*He will prepare the people for the coming of the Lord. He will turn the hearts of the fathers to their children*' (NLT)

We all know that family life doesn't always run smoothly. We've probably all experienced arguments at home to some degree, and sometimes deeply ingrained problems can lead to relationships within families completely breaking down. But, even when problems at home seem really out of hand, God can heal the rifts and bring family members back together. Sometimes we need a mediator to help us sort things out in a calm and controlled way, and sometimes professional intervention is the best course of action – but we can always pray, and the Church can be enormously supportive in healing broken relationships within families.

What an amazing prophecy for Zechariah to hear about his unborn son. John the Baptist's ministry would be all about reconciliation – bringing people closer to God and to each other. A hallmark of God's work through John was parents being reconciled to their sons and daughters. Our God is the same God who reconciles, and He can make us peacemakers too. In His strength, difficult situations in our families can be turned around. He longs to redeem what has been broken, and restore what has been lost.

Pray
Ask God to heal rifts in any family you know that is having problems. If this is your own family, talk to a close friend you trust and ask them to pray, too.

Weekend

21/22 SEP

Take care

READ: 1 TIMOTHY 5:1–16

KEY VERSE V4
'their first responsibility is to show godliness at home and repay their parents by taking care of them.' (NLT)

The Bible is clear on how we need to treat those older than us with the respect they deserve. Getting older is part of life – and Proverbs even describes grey hair as 'the splendour of the old' (Prov. 20:29)! However, old age isn't always particularly glamorous. Our bodies eventually start to shut down, and we'll find that we need help with our mobility, memory, and perhaps even the most basic tasks. Perhaps your grandparents (or maybe even your parents, depending on how old you are) are getting towards that stage now. This isn't meant to sound morbid – growing old is a very natural process – but the simple fact

is that we are required to care for the elderly
when they need our help.

We all have a God-given responsibility to
look after our family members, whatever age
they are. Today's Bible passage gives some clear
advice to those of us who are younger and able-
bodied that it is our responsibility to take care
of the vulnerable members of our families. And
don't forget the importance of emotional care.
Even if you have relatives who don't need much
practical help, never underestimate the impact
of some quality time spent with them.

 ## Challenge

*What one or two practical things can you do to
help those in your family? Maybe you could help
with housework or say encouraging words more
often. Whatever you think of, commit to doing it
this week.*

At all times

READ: PROVERBS 17:17–22

KEY VERSE V17
'A friend is always loyal, and a brother is born to help in time of need.' (NLT)

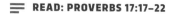

Do you have brothers and sisters? How well do you get on with them? Our relationship with our siblings can be the trickiest of all. Maybe you're fighting like cat and dog one minute, and the next minute you're the best of friends, laughing your heads off!

We all get on each other's nerves sometimes – even the 'super Christian' families. But the point is, we're called to have each other's backs. When things get tough, family members (and friends) need help and support from each other. We're not designed to go it alone, and there's no time you'll ever need your friends more than 'in time of need'.

The other thing this passage points out is that 'a friend is always loyal'. In the NIV, it says 'A friend loves at all times' (v17). *All times* – not just when we're having a nice time, or it's in our own interest. We need to love people, even when they're being a massive pain. We need to remain loyal to those in our family, especially when we don't feel like it.

Are you going through a tough time at the moment? Ask God for the right people to help you out. Is there someone in your family, your friendship group or your church who needs a 'brother' to 'help in time of need' right now? Maybe you can be that person!

HOT TOPIC | FAMILY 1

➕ *Challenge*
Think about how you can support someone you love this week, whether practically or emotionally.

God provides

≡ **READ: 1 KINGS 17:8–24**

KEY VERSE V9
'Go at once to Zarephath in the region of Sidon and stay there. I have directed a widow there to supply you with food.'

In today's world, 'family' doesn't always mean mum, dad and 2.4 kids. For example, a lot of families include just one parent, either because the parents have separated or, as in the case of the woman in today's reading, because one parent has died. Parenting and providing can be hard work – even more so when you're doing it solo.

The family in today's reading had an extremely tough time. Not only was the father of the family dead, but they had to survive through a famine without him. But through Elijah, amazingly, miraculously, God blesses the woman and her son. God always provides enough food for them and even brings the son back to life when he dies!

There may be pain and difficulties in single parent families, but God can and does bless families in this situation. Perhaps you can identify with the family in 1 Kings 17. Perhaps your family is struggling; perhaps it even feels like you're totally without hope. If so, God is still with you. Whatever form your family takes, whatever struggles you face, however bleak things may seem, God can still make amazing things happen.

HOT TOPIC | FAMILY 1

↑ *Pray*

God, You are my provider. You are the one who raises the dead. You are the one who brings hope. Thank You that You are with my family, whatever happens. I commit them to You now. Amen.

Spiritual parents

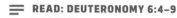

READ: DEUTERONOMY 6:4–9

KEY VERSE V7
'Repeat [these commands] again and again to your children.' (NLT)

Have you been brought up in a Christian family? Did you get taken along to church and Sunday school as a child, and get tucked up at night with a Bible reading and a bedtime prayer? Or have you come to know Jesus because of the input of someone else, who has shown you what it means to live for Jesus and encouraged you in your own walk with Him?

As we've been discovering, none of us are supposed to go it alone on the Christian journey. We need community (and what we call 'fellowship' with other Christians) in a family of fellow believers. The foundations laid in our early days of faith are really important. If there are Christians in your family, make the most of their wisdom, experience and support. If you're the only Christian in your family, you can find spiritual 'parents' in your church – older Christians who can offer you their support and guidance (it's always helpful to have figures like this in your life outside of your own family as well anyway!). And even now you can start making decisions about the kind of spiritual parent you want to be in the future – how one day you can support your own kids (or other people's kids) in their faith in Jesus.

HOT TOPIC | FAMILY 1

Think

How are you getting on with God at the moment? Are you struggling with anything? How can your family or your spiritual 'parents' help you?

In good times and bad

READ: ROMANS 12:9–21

KEY VERSE V15
'Be happy with those who are happy, and weep with those who weep.' (NLT)

HOT TOPIC | FAMILY 1

The Simpsons have a lot to teach us. They're by no means a perfect family. (In fact, maybe it's the characters' quirks and faults that make them likeable and realistic.) Bart and Lisa are constantly at each other's throats and Homer's relationship with his dad is famously awkward. But, underneath all this, the family are deeply committed to each other. When something goes well, they share each other's joy. When one of them is suffering, all the other family members rally around to support them. When Homer finds fame as an astronaut, for example, his family celebrate with him. When he is falsely accused of a crime, they stand by him.

Of course, the Simpsons are a fictional caricature of what family life can be like, but perhaps this is how God wants us to treat our families! In Romans 12, the apostle Paul lists some very important qualities in family life and church life alike, and underpinning it all is a deep commitment to our relatives. This means being there for them in the good times and sticking with them in the bad times. Share their joy when things are great and cry with them when it all goes wrong. When we do that, the annoying little niggles don't seem to matter quite as much.

 Challenge

Choose to love your family and commit yourself to them, whatever happens. This won't always be easy, so ask for God's strength to do this.

Jesus' family tree

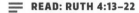

READ: RUTH 4:13–22

KEY VERSE V17
'And they named him Obed. He was the father of Jesse, the father of David.'

Who'd have thought it? A Moabite – a refugee and an enemy of the Jews – turns out to be an ancestor of King David, and even an ancestor of Jesus Himself! Ruth wasn't particularly special in herself, but because of her faithfulness to God and to her family, God was able to use her for something extraordinary – and Jesus ended up being born into that family line, and part of that family tree! How special is that!

We might not think our families are anything special. When we live with people, it's easy to see their faults and annoying habits. It's much harder to see their good points. It's harder still to see their potential – what they could do and become. Sometimes it's harder when we *don't* live with people! But God can do amazing things through ordinary people and ordinary families, through their faithfulness to God and to each other. We might not see the results now – maybe not even in our lifetime – but God blesses families and can do amazing things through them. So, as we end this first section of our studies on Family, remember this: keep loving your relatives. Stay committed to them and to God, and some brilliant things can happen.

HOT TOPIC | FAMILY 1

🕱 *Think*

Try to look at your family members as if you were meeting them for the first time. What good qualities do they have? Think and pray about what God could accomplish through your family.

**WEEKEND
28/29 SEP**

CELEBRATE

Rollercoaster ride

READ: ECCLESIASTES 3:1–8

KEY VERSE V4
'A time to weep and a time to laugh,
a time to mourn and a time to dance'

Welcome to the first part of our look at celebrating!
We've got some great times ahead of us as we get
into why, how and when we celebrate, and what the
Bible says about all this.

Our lives are made up of so many different
experiences and emotions. Unless you are a robot,
you may have already experienced some incredibly
dizzy highs and possibly also some deep, dark lows
in your life. We all experience a variety of emotions,
and sometimes, we might feel like we're on an
emotional rollercoaster.

The passage from Ecclesiastes expands this simple fact of life for us. It tells us that we will probably not dance our way through every single part of life – there will be times when we don't want to celebrate. Times when life gets tough. But our key verse reminds us that these don't last forever, and we'll see times worth celebrating again.

Good times and celebrations are part of life. God set it up that way, as you'll see. Sometimes, as Christians, we think our faith is so serious that we walk around with scrunched up faces, stepping away from anything that looks fun. Our faith *is* serious – it's a life-or-death kind of issue – but it's also absolutely fantastic, amazing and worth celebrating! Life is worth celebrating too – as well as all the good things God has created for us.

We can learn from all the different times we go through in life – both the sad times and the happy times – but remember that we will again see times for a good old party!

Think

What celebrations have you taken part in during the last year? Birthdays? Family events? Parties? Have a think about what these celebrations looked like, what you enjoyed about them, and if there's anything you'd do differently now.

The life of the party

READ: JOHN 2:1–10

KEY VERSE V2

'Jesus and his disciples had also been invited to the wedding.'

Do you think Jesus approves of partying? Judging from today's reading, it seems He didn't only go to parties – He brought the party! We learnt yesterday that there should be times of celebration in our lives and Jesus' actions at this wedding show just how high a priority this is.

First of all, Jesus goes to the wedding party. Although it's important to follow Jesus' example of taking some time away from others, for just us and God to spend together (which Jesus did on many occasions), it's equally important to learn from His life that hanging out with others and enjoying their company is good, and is actually a God-given thing to do.

Secondly, when Jesus miraculously turns the water into wine, He makes it the best they've ever tasted! Jesus doesn't give them supermarket own brand wine so that they'll hate it and go home; He seems to have wanted people to stay and enjoy themselves. That's not to say that Jesus wanted everyone to get drunk; Luke 21:34 shows us that he's not in favour of that. But what we can see here is that Jesus enjoyed life and He loved seeing other people enjoy themselves too!

Challenge

Sometimes we accept a view of Jesus that isn't actually what He is like. Write down some lies that people often believe about Jesus. Then, cross through them with a line and underneath write down the truth about Him.

HOT TOPIC | CELEBRATE 1

Sunday funday

READ: EXODUS 20:8–11

KEY VERSE V11
'the Lᴏʀᴅ blessed the Sabbath day and made it holy.'

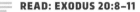

When God created the world, He set rhythm at the heart of it. Seasons come and seasons go, the moon directs our months and our hearts beat rhythmically until the day we die. God set within us a need to rest regularly, and He gave us a weekly model when He created the world – on the seventh day, He rested.

The word 'Sabbath' literally means to cease. The Jews were told to cease working one day a week (sundown Friday to sundown Saturday). It wasn't just nice advice that God gave, or His 'top tip' for surviving as a human: it was a command. God knows that this is what we need. How great is that? Even when our lives are crazily busy, even when we're up to our eyeballs in work, God wants us to take a day out.

As Christians, most of us tend to celebrate the Lord's Day on Sundays – to celebrate and remember Jesus' resurrection. We don't have strict rules because for some people (for example, shift workers) their day of rest might not be a Sunday. But the principle remains: once a week we need to stop and spend time with God, relax and unwind from the week, and celebrate together with our friends and family. What an incredible command!

 Pray
Father, help me to get into the habit of spending one day every week resting and celebrating, and getting closer to You. Amen.

HOT TOPIC | CELEBRATE 1

Festival tickets

READ: EXODUS 23:14–16

KEY VERSE V14
'Three times a year you are to celebrate a festival to me.'

HOT TOPIC | CELEBRATE 1

Yesterday, we learnt that God calls (even commands) us to a weekly time of rest. In today's passage, God puts some dates in the Israelites' diaries for their yearly celebrations. As Israel grew as a nation, more festivals were added to these three, but these were the original ones.

All three festivals were set times to remember God and to celebrate Him. In the Festival of Unleavened Bread, the Israelites were to remember how God had brought them out of Egypt and to celebrate His goodness in doing so. In the two harvest festivals, they remembered how God had created everything to be enjoyed, and they celebrated God for giving them food for survival.

We don't celebrate the festivals set out in Exodus, but as Christians we've got plenty of events to celebrate throughout the year: the biggies – Christmas and Easter – but also others like Palm Sunday, Pentecost and Advent. Each festival is there for us to remember and celebrate God – He knows that we need yearly reminders of the good things He has done for us.

 ## *Challenge*
It's still a few months until Christmas, but why not get prepared and think of ways to remember who it's all about in the midst of the decorations, gifts and festivities. You could set some reminders in your phone to remind you of these things to do during December to celebrate Jesus coming to earth.

VIP

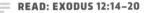

READ: EXODUS 12:14–20

KEY VERSE V14
'Each year, from generation to generation, you must celebrate it as a special festival to the LORD.' (NLT)

Carrying on our theme of celebrating and remembering, this passage is specifically about the Festival of Unleavened Bread, and the instructions in the passage are actually given before the Israelites have left Egypt. The words seem a little strong, even harsh. What's the big deal about yeast, anyway?

The big deal for Israel, the reason why God so desperately wanted His people to remember it, was for them to remember *who* they were and *whose* they were. If at any point they were to forget these, once the Festival of Unleavened Bread came around in the springtime it would all become clear again: 'Oh yes, I'm an Israelite, loved so much by God who rescued us out of Egypt.'

Do your celebrations remind you of who you are in Christ? Taking a Sabbath, a day of rest, should remind you that your value is not in what you do or achieve, but in who you are. Celebrating Easter will help you remember that you are saved through Jesus' death on the cross. Christmas tells you that God loved you enough to become human and that He knows what it's like to experience life as a human being. God's celebrations show that you are a VIP, a *very* important person.

HOT TOPIC | CELEBRATE 1

 Pray
Lord, please help me remember who I am today, that I am loved by You, set free by You and made whole by You. Help me be reminded of my identity in You through the times when I celebrate who You are and what You've done. Amen.

Credit where credit's due

READ: EXODUS 32:1–21

KEY VERSE V19
'When Moses approached the camp and saw the calf and the dancing, his anger burned'

Although we can see that God is up for a good party and has even created festivals for us, He is very specific about what should be celebrated and what should not. God had the right idea when He set up those festivals we've been reading about as reminders to Israel, because, in today's passage, they have completely forgotten who they are and what they are all about as a nation.

It might be hard for us to understand how the Israelites could forget that it was God who had led them out of Egypt, and instead give the praise for their rescue to a golden calf. But let's be honest with ourselves: we can act very similarly.

Do you ever forget who saved you? Do you ever forget about God and start celebrating idols? You probably don't literally bow down to things like a golden calf, but we might bow our hearts down to other things – giving them all our attention and praise, and ignoring God. Maybe it's a band, celebrity, clothes, or even your games console. None of these things are necessarily wrong to enjoy, but if we start celebrating them in God's place, that's when it becomes a problem.

Think

Do you ever find yourself caring less about God and getting more excited about other things or people instead? Do you think you ever celebrate idols? If you need to say sorry and make some changes, do so – then remember: He loves you and forgives you immediately.

Weekend

5/6 OCT

Flashmob!

READ: EXODUS 15:1–21

KEY VERSE V21
'Sing to the LORD, for he has triumphed gloriously; he has hurled both horse and rider into the sea.' (NLT)

Have you ever seen God do something so amazing that you couldn't stop yourself from bursting into spontaneous song? If you are the kind of person that loves to write worship songs to praise God, then you're in good company because here's an original from Moses and Miriam – complete with the rest of the Israelites on backing vocals and, of course, a tambourine.

Can you imagine the scene? You have just seen a sea – yes, a large mass of water – divide in two to allow you through. That's mind-blowing! It's easy to see where Moses got his inspiration from, and he quickly begins to get the band together and praises God as his 'strength', his 'song', a 'warrior', 'glorious in power', 'glorious in holiness', 'awesome in splendour'. Wow – what a fantastic celebration of who God is! This makes your average worship song look like a nursery rhyme.

So again, what about you? When have you been really excited about something God's done? You might think He's not done anything for you like He did for Moses, but wait a minute. Take a step back and look. He's done so many incredible things for you, more than can be counted, but here's some highlights: He has adopted you into His family (Eph. 1:5), He has died for you (Rom. 5:8), He has forgiven you (Eph. 1:7), He has saved you (1 Thess. 5:9) and He has promised to always be with you (Matt. 28:20).

This really is the sort of stuff worth celebrating – the goodness of our God has just got to be celebrated!

 ## Challenge

Have a go at writing your own song, poem or rap to celebrate God for who He is and what He has done. You can start afresh, rewrite Moses' song into your own words or use other Bible verses to inspire you.

Sound the trumpets!

READ: 2 CHRONICLES 5:7–14

KEY VERSE V13
'The trumpeters and musicians joined in unison to give praise and thanks to the LORD.'

We've taken a look at remembering God, celebrating Him and not celebrating idols, but here is the ultimate example of an all-out 'God celebration'!

This passage is all about the moving of the Ark of the Covenant into the newly built Temple, and it was a pretty huge deal. It was an incredibly exciting and important event for Israel, because both the Temple and the Ark in some ways symbolised God's presence with them as a nation. So, the people going a bit crazy in this passage were not doing it because they were obsessed with some religious monuments, but because God was near!

Imagine 120 trumpeters together with all sorts of other instruments – that would have created quite a sound! They were not holding back at all; they gave it everything. And God joined in with the celebrations by covering the crowds as a thick cloud.

How often are we this extravagant in our celebration of God? He deserves the very best we've got. We might not be able to get our hands on 120 trumpets, but there are definitely other ways that we can go all-out in our praise for God.

HOT TOPIC | CELEBRATE 1

Think

How can you celebrate God extravagantly today? Maybe you could organise a worship evening with your friends (or ask your leader to organise one), create a piece of art, or even share something about God on your social media.

Bring and share

READ: NEHEMIAH 8:5–12

KEY VERSE V12
'So the people went away... to celebrate with great joy because they had heard God's words and understood them.' (NLT)

Who has ever heard of a sermon so good that it kick-started a full-blown celebration, including food, drinks and gifts? Sounds impossible, but this is pretty much what happened in today's passage.

The book of Nehemiah tells the story of the people of Israel returning to their land after having been captive in Babylon for 400 years. They had lost almost everything: material possessions, their dignity and, in some ways, their identity. Do you remember how important it was for Israel to remember who they were?

To help them remember, Ezra, who was a scribe and a priest, read 'the Law' to the whole people. ('The Law' doesn't just mean a list of commands, but the first five books of the Bible.) And they started to remember! At first the people began to mourn, perhaps because they realised what they had lost and forgotten. But Ezra told them that this was not the way to react to God's Word. The proper response was to celebrate! They were the only nation in the world to have been given the Law – that was a huge privilege. So what did they do? They celebrated in the obvious Christian way: a bring and share lunch! God's Word was – and still is today – worth celebrating.

 Pray
Heavenly Father, thank You that many of us have freedom to own and read Your Word. Help me to never take that for granted. Amen.

HOT TOPIC | CELEBRATE 1

No filter

READ:2 SAMUEL 6:12–23

KEY VERSE V22
*'Yes, and I am willing to look even more foolish than
this, even to be humiliated in my own eyes!' (NLT)*

In most societies, huge emphasis is placed on image.
People get so hung up on having the 'perfect' image
(whatever that is) and showing it off to the world. So how
does that affect the way we celebrate God? Do you ever
feel like you need to downplay your celebration of who
God is in order to keep up your image?

This isn't just a question we face today, it's something
that God's people have always had to address. David's
wife, Michal, clearly believed the lie that image was
everything. She might have been powerful and married to
the king, but God knew how hard her heart was. David, on
the other hand, who God calls 'a man after my own heart'
(Acts 13:22), didn't care about what other people thought,
but allowed himself to be caught up in the celebrations.

The Temple and the Ark of the Covenant, symbolised the
presence of God. David was celebrating, going for it and not
letting anyone's embarrassment stop him, because God
had drawn near. He didn't care that he looked ridiculous;
he was willing to be even more humiliated, as long as it
was for, and in true worship of, the God he loved.

HOT TOPIC | CELEBRATE 1

Think
*Are there things you choose not to do because you fear
damaging your image? Why not aim to be like David and
openly celebrate the fact that God loves you.*

Beyond the singing

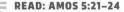

READ: AMOS 5:21–24

KEY VERSE V21
'I hate, I despise your religious festivals; your assemblies are a stench to me.'

Hold up! What's going on here? All of a sudden God hates the festivals? These verses might come as a surprise after all we've read about God's festivals and how important they were for Israel's identity. But God had good reason to hate the specific festivals being spoken about here.

In about 760 BC, Amos was sent by God from Judah, the southern kingdom, to Israel, the northern kingdom (the two kingdoms having split in about 926 BC). Neither kingdom escapes criticism in Amos' powerful prophecy, but it's the Israelites who get the worse deal. Their failure is summed up in verse 24: they had forgotten about justice and righteousness. They have kept their religious festivals, done all the singing and sacrificing by the book, while treating the poor in their society like dirt.

Jesus had a special love for the poor and, very much like Amos, had some strong words to say to religious people who forgot about justice. It is not hard to imagine how God feels when we throw yet another praise party but make the homeless person feel unwelcome in church. Of course God wants to be celebrated, but caring for the people He has created and loves is a huge part of our worship.

✚ *Challenge*

How can your church or youth group do more to bring justice to the world? Think of a way in which you can do some 'justice worship' on top of the usual 'singing worship'. Bring the suggestion to a church leader.

HOT TOPIC | CELEBRATE 1

Praise the Lord

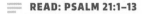

READ: PSALM 21:1–13

KEY VERSE V13
'With music and singing we celebrate your mighty acts.' (NLT)

As we come to the end of the first part of our look at celebrating, we read a psalm that really spells out just how great God is and why He is worth celebrating. David, pen in hand, is composing another psalm – a worship song – jotting down some of the reasons why he personally wants to celebrate God.

First, he gets excited about who God is: He is strong (v1) and has unfailing love (v7). Then, David celebrates what God has done for him: He has granted him his desires (v2), blessed him (v3) and given him victories (v5). Towards the end of the psalm, David shows just how powerful God is in dealing with those who try to bring God down. And then he wraps it up with a great declaration of worship.

We have learnt over the last couple of weeks that God is up for celebrations – big time! He is the one we should celebrate – He's absolutely incredible and so are the things He does for us.

Coming up in part two of 'Celebrate', along with some top tips from the Early Church about celebration, there's more great news: God celebrates us! But until then, let's remember to celebrate the one who deserves it all.

HOT TOPIC | CELEBRATE 1

Pray
Father, I thank You for all Your mighty acts. Thank You for how You have acted in my life just in these last couple of weeks. I celebrate You now for Your goodness. Help me to maintain an attitude of celebration in all I do. Amen.

**WEEKEND
12/13 OCT**

INTEGRITY

It's a promise
READ: GENESIS 39:1–23

KEY VERSE V8
'But he refused. "With me in charge," he told her, "my master does not concern himself with anything in the house."'

Trust is something that is not given lightly. Over time, we may trust people once we have seen evidence of them keeping their word or not passing on anything that has been told them in confidence. When we trust someone, we make ourselves vulnerable to them and rely on them to stick to their promises. The same principle applies to ourselves. Keeping a promise or being true to *our* word is how we can show people that we have integrity. With this thought, we begin our journey to discover what integrity really is and how we can learn to live lives of integrity.

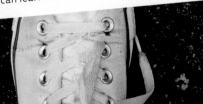

In today's reading, we see that Joseph has integrity. Sold as a slave, Joseph is initially given small tasks to do. When he proves totally trustworthy and successful in these, he is made Potiphar's personal attendant. God continues to give Joseph success in everything he does, so he is trusted with more and more. In verses 7–8, we see Joseph's trustworthiness and integrity tested. Potiphar's wife wants to sleep with him but he knows it would betray his master's trust, and would also be acting unfaithfully towards God. He refuses. Having integrity is important to Joseph; he keeps his integrity in everything he does, no matter what the cost to himself.

Proverbs 11:20 tells us that God 'delights in those with integrity'. In everything we do, we should seek to live as God wants us to, with integrity – just like Joseph. When people around us look at the way we live, they should be able to see something different about us: that we stick to what we say and keep our promises.

Think

As we start to look at the topic of integrity, think about what it means to you. Are there people you know who are living lives of integrity? What is different about them? Where in your life do you need to exercise more integrity?

Practise what you preach

READ: 2 SAMUEL 12:1–10

KEY VERSE V7
'Then Nathan said to David, "You are that man!"'

In the UK and most countries, the legal age to vote is 18 years old. Voting is a great opportunity to voice your opinion about what happens in local and national politics. You can influence who is in government and have some say about decisions that can affect your future. This is a sentiment promoted by the celebrity Paris Hilton. She famously encouraged young Americans to vote in 2004. Later, however, it was revealed that not only did Paris Hilton fail to vote herself but that she had not registered to vote!

Have you heard the saying: 'Practise what you preach'? It means to put into practice yourself, the things you tell others to do – exactly what Paris Hilton failed to do. In today's reading, David learns a similar lesson.

God made David king of Israel to uphold justice and lead the people, but, sadly, David didn't maintain that justice in his own personal life. God sent Nathan the prophet to rebuke him for murdering Uriah after sleeping with Uriah's wife. David was a great king – but this lack of integrity led to God's intervention. In a world full of hypocrisy, we need to be people who practise what we preach. Before making bold declarations, let's make sure we maintain those principles ourselves.

Pray

Lord, help me to put into practice the things I preach and to think about my own lifestyle before commenting on the lives of others. Amen.

HOT TOPIC | INTEGRITY 1

When no one's watching...

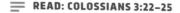

READ: COLOSSIANS 3:22–25

KEY VERSE V22
'Try to please them all the time, not just when they are watching you.' (NLT)

A research programme on television recently tested the honesty of young children. One by one, each child was taken into a room. The teacher told them not to look in the box placed on a table in front of them. While the teacher was in the room, the children followed the instruction but, as soon as the teacher left, these five-year-olds could not resist a little peek. When the teacher returned, the children were asked whether they had looked in the box. Each child answered 'No'. Unknown to them, secret cameras in the room had been recording their actions and so revealed the truth.

Perhaps we wouldn't be tricked as easily as these five-year-olds. However, do we act as if we are being watched? Do we remember that God sees *all* our actions? Have we become used to telling people we live a certain way, only to act differently?

Our reading challenges us to work hard and live with integrity all the time – not just when others are watching us. By following this advice, we are actually doing ourselves a favour by gaining a reputation of being responsible young adults who can be left to work independently.

HOT TOPIC | INTEGRITY 1

➕ Challenge

Throughout today, think about your actions as if others could see you. You may find that you are making different choices.

Get back on track

READ: PSALM 15:1–5

KEY VERSE V3
'Those who refuse to gossip or harm their neighbors or speak evil of their friends.' (NLT)

HOT TOPIC | INTEGRITY 1

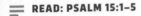

Have you ever had to write a CV or a record of achievement statement? It involves having to list everything you've done and the attributes that make you employable. Or perhaps you have filled out an application form for a job? Again, you need to write about your strengths and what makes you suitable for the job. When the employers look through the CVs and job application forms, they want to know whether you fit the job description.

Fortunately for us, God doesn't choose us based on our CVs or on how good an application form we write to become a Christian. Nevertheless, we do find descriptions in the Bible of how God wants us to live. We can also look at how Jesus lived as an example of living the best way.

Today's reading demonstrates how God longs for His people to live lives of integrity: living blamelessly, doing what is right, speaking the truth, having sincere hearts and not insulting others. If we mess up and don't live this way, we don't lose our jobs or become unfit to be a Christian. However, we do stop living the way God has planned for us. Let's get back on track, put bad habits behind us and get on board with God's guidelines for how to live.

 ## *Challenge*
Would you be able to fit the job description from today's reading? If there is anything you need to change and behave differently, talk to God about it, seek His forgiveness and make a fresh start today.

Hair model

READ: PROVERBS 10:6–11

KEY VERSE V9
'People with integrity walk safely, but those who follow crooked paths will be exposed.' (NLT)

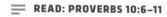

Who do you admire? Your parents? A musician? A politician? A teacher? A football player? What is it about them that is so admirable? What is it about the way they live their lives?

Many people admire celebrities for their confidence or their abilities in a chosen field. Other people may be admired for sticking to their beliefs or for the way they treat those around them.

One admirable person is a young boy from Florida called Christian McPhilamy. At the age of six, he decided to grow his hair for two years before having it cut and created into wigs for children with hair loss. It wasn't an easy thing to do and severally people bullied him about his long blonde hair. Even some adults suggested that he should get a haircut. But he stuck it out, and didn't stray from his goal. Eventually, after two years, Christian had grown over 10 inches of hair to be donated to a charity.

Ask yourself: why do you admire a certain person? Is it because of what they can do or have? Or is it because of how they act – with integrity? If an eight-year-old boy can do something to help and inspire others, maybe you too could be an inspiration to those around you.

HOT TOPIC | INTEGRITY 1

Think

What is it about you that others find admirable? Take time to think about who you are a role model to and how you can live a life of integrity.

A tough test for Job

READ: JOB 27:1–6

KEY VERSE V6
'I will maintain my innocence without wavering. My conscience is clear for as long as I live.' (NLT)

HOT TOPIC | INTEGRITY 1

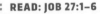

Have you read the book of Job? It's a challenging but fascinating story. It's about Job's faithfulness to God being tested by the devil when everything is taken from him. But Job keeps his integrity and chooses never to curse God.

All his farm animals are stolen and farmhands killed, his sheep are burnt up along with their shepherds, his camels are stolen and his servants killed. Job's sons and daughters are all killed by a collapsing house and he is struck with a severe case of boils all over his body. Throughout all his sufferings, his friends accuse him of sinning. All in all, not a great time for old Job.

Job refuses to believe that this suffering is due to sin as he has always remained faithful to God. He claims his conscience is completely clear. And he's right. It was not sin that caused these afflictions but a test of his integrity.

Job's wife urges him to curse God and to give up on life so that he will die and the sufferings will stop. However, Job refuses and says nothing wrong against God. He remains faithful to God – even when others wrongly say he would be justified in blaming God. Job lives his life with integrity through the good times *and* the bad.

➕ Challenge
Would you be able to stand up for your beliefs in good times and bad? How much integrity do you show in your relationship with God when others come and challenge you?

Weekend

19/20 OCT

Live in harmony
READ: ROMANS 14:1–4

≡ KEY VERSE V2
'For instance, one person believes it's all right to eat anything.' (NLT)

What do you think is the difference between morals and conscience? Well, morals are standards of right and wrong behavior, whereas a conscience is a sense of right and wrong that helps govern our thoughts and actions. Both work together to help us to make good choices.

Many of our morals may be exactly like those of people around us; for example, that killing and stealing are wrong. Other morals are more personal and may be based on how we have been brought up; for instance, we may choose to only eat Fair Trade chocolate. Our morals tell us what is right and wrong, but our view of right and wrong may not be the same as that of the next person.

Paul addressed a church that struggled with the issue of differing morals. Some felt it was not right to eat certain meats, others felt it was OK. Both had a compelling argument. Paul does not give an answer to set them all straight once and for all, but teaches them to live in harmony with their differences, since some differences are acceptable.

While we might not agree with them, it is good to be aware that other people might have a different set of morals to ourselves.

Pray

Ask God to give you wisdom and insight into your own morals. Ask Him to show you which standards and beliefs are good, and how you can live with those around you who don't share the same views.

Defending what's right

READ: NEHEMIAH 4:10–14

KEY VERSE V14
'Remember the Lord, who is great and awesome, and fight for your families... and your homes.'

There are plenty of 'Your mum' jokes on the internet or you may have heard some of them. When they are said in jest, they might seem very funny. But imagine if people were saying unkind things about your mum, dad or relative, and they were serious. You would probably feel that they were being very disrespectful towards your family. You might even get very angry and let that person know that what they are saying is totally out of order. This urge to defend your family might be stronger than the urge to defend any jokes directed at yourself. Most of us want to look out for our families. Nevertheless, we also need to balance that with the moral that fighting is wrong, and that it's not up to us to take revenge.

Our morals tell us what is right: that our loved ones come first. Nehemiah commanded the Israelites to defend what was important: their friends, family and homes. He loved the people and was willing to be their leader and to fight to protect them. If he had not believed that families were important, his command might have been: 'Every man for himself!' However, even in battle, family, friends and homes remained important.

Pray

Thank God for your family and friends. Ask for God's help to value them and stand up for them in appropriate ways, and for the strength to turn your back on things you know are wrong.

HOT TOPIC | INTEGRITY 1

Against the norm

 READ: 1 PETER 2:9–12

KEY VERSE V12
'though they accuse you of doing wrong, they may see your good deeds and glorify God'

Daniel was an Old Testament Bible character who was taken into exile from Jerusalem to Babylon. Clever and healthy young men were particularly selected to work in the king's palace. There were to be trained for three years, and were given food and wine to drink. Daniel and some of his close friends, however, decided to abstain from this royal food and wine and at the end of ten days 'looked healthier and better nourished than any of the young men who ate the royal food' (Dan. 1:15).

Most of us will probably have good friends who are not Christians or don't believe in God. It's great to have these friends – but we also need to be true to what we believe and to what our morals tell us. In an effort to fit in with our friends or to be culturally relevant, we can end up compromising what we believe.

It's important to live honourable lives so that our non-Christian friends will see our behaviour and respect our actions. We don't have to do whatever our friends tell us to do; neither is it a good idea to let our behaviour affect our relationship with God. You might lose some friendships by sticking to your morals, but you might also develop some closer and deeper friendships from those that respect you.

 ## *Think*

Where do you need to be true to your morals despite what others might say? Take a stand and be prepared to go against the norm.

No compromise

READ: EXODUS 32:1–8

KEY VERSE V4
'Then Aaron took the gold, melted it down, and moulded it into the shape of a calf.' (NLT)

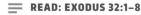

After leaving Egypt, where they had been enslaved for many years, the Israelites wandered around in the desert wilderness. They were refugees with no land to call their home. They made camp while Moses, their leader, was away on Mount Sinai talking with God. Moses had been absent for a long time and the Israelite people were getting restless. The Egyptians and other neighbouring countries had their own man-made gods, which they were able to worship, so why couldn't they? Aaron, Moses' brother, fell for their argument. In wanting to please the people and keep the peace, he gave in to their demands and fashioned an image of a god in the form of a golden calf for them to worship

Perhaps Aaron thought, 'How bad can it be? Other people are doing it.' Or maybe he understood their desire to fit in with others. However good (or otherwise) his intentions may have been, he compromised his integrity and his morals. Without the support of his brother, Moses, he might have felt weaker and unable to stand firm against the people.

Our intentions may be good, but we must make sure that we never lower or compromise our morals or beliefs for the sake of pleasing others or fitting in.

HOT TOPIC | INTEGRITY 1

➕ **Challenge**

Have you compromised your beliefs? What do you need to rethink or do differently so they are not compromised again?

Be bold, be strong

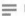

READ: ROMANS 2:6–16

KEY VERSE V15
'their own conscience and thoughts either accuse them or tell them they are doing right.' (NLT)

HOT TOPIC | INTEGRITY 1

Adam and Eve – one couple that took eating their five-a-day to the extreme! God had told them not to eat the fruit on one of the trees. But, one day, Eve was walking past that beautiful tree and the fruit was looking so tempting, ripe and juicy. Surely, it couldn't hurt to have a little taste? God wouldn't want her to miss out on something so delicious, would He? Even the snake agreed with her that God couldn't possible cause her to die after carefully creating her. 'So she took some of the fruit and ate it' (Gen. 1:6). Then Eve gave some to Adam as well. Suddenly, they knew what they had done was wrong and tried to hide from God.

Our conscience and our morals help us to know when things are wrong without us being told. When young, we learn from our parents what is right and wrong and we often hear the word 'no'. As we grow up, we have our conscience (an intrinsic part of us put there by God) that knows right from wrong without being told. We need to listen to our conscience and keep our integrity. Sometimes, when we know we are straying off the right path, we need to say 'no' to ourselves. What do you need to do to keep you away from something you know, deep in your heart, is wrong?

Pray

Ask for God's guidance in those times when it's difficult to know what is right and what is wrong, strength to enable you to have the willpower to say 'no' and boldness to go a different way.

On a journey to truth

READ: JOB 10:8–12

KEY VERSE V10
'You guided my conception and formed me in the womb.' (NLT)

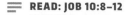

Each one of us has been conceived and formed in a womb. We have all started life as an embryo and then formed major organs, nerves, muscles and skin – all while still inside our mother's womb. We were each given the gift of life and are all loved by God.

Once born, we each have very different lives. We have different parents or carers, different homes and different educations. Our paths in life are unique and shape us into the people we are today. This will inevitably mean that we have different thoughts on what we believe and why.

We may think that our beliefs are right and that everyone else is wrong, that we have it all sorted and that others need to think the same way as us. However, until we see God, no one can be certain they have everything right. We cannot know everything there is to know about God while we are on this earth. Each one of us still has things to learn.

With this in mind, we need to be careful not to judge others because they don't believe what we believe. Instead, let the way we act point people to the good things about Jesus. As Christians, we believe that we have found the way, the truth and the life in Jesus Christ. Other people haven't got there yet, just be patient and pray for them.

HOT TOPIC | INTEGRITY 1

Think

How can you be tolerant and love others who don't share the same beliefs?

THE BIBLE

Hot off the press?

READ: ISAIAH 40:3–8

KEY VERSE V8
'the word of our God endures for ever.'

Shakespeare is probably the world's most famous playwright. There are millions of copies of Shakespeare's plays but there is only one surviving handwritten script in existence. Three pages of a manuscript, written sometime between 1601 and 1604, are safely archived in the British Library. As the Bible was written between 1450 BC and AD 96, way before Shakespeare, it is not surprising that there are no original manuscripts of the Bible in existence. So how do we know that the Bible is authentic?

Well, although there are no original manuscripts, there are copies. The oldest complete copy of the Old Testament is in a museum in St Petersburg, Russia and is dated AD 1000. This is still a long time after the originals were written, which is why some wondered if they were the original words.

Then, in 1947, some well-preserved fragments of manuscripts were found by shepherds in caves near the Dead Sea. These Dead Sea Scrolls, as they were called, dated back to 100 BC and contained parts of the Old Testament. When these were compared to later copies of the Old Testament, they were virtually the same.

Isaiah's prophecy reminds us that even though seasons changes, years roll on and time passes, the 'word of our God endures for ever' (v8). The Bible has taken various forms over the centuries: verbally passed on from person to person, written on manuscripts, printed books and digital formats. But whatever physical form the Bible has taken, the words it contains are hugely powerful and have conveyed the most important fact of all: God loves us.

Challenge

Why not Google 'Dead Sea Scrolls' and 'Leningrad Codex' to learn more information about these very old manuscripts?

A glimpse into the future

≡ **READ: ISAIAH 52:13–15; 53:1–12**

KEY VERSE 53:7
'He was oppressed and afflicted, yet he did not open his mouth; he was led like a lamb to the slaughter.'

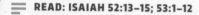

'By the rivers of Babylon, where we sat down, yeah we wept, when we remembered Zion. When the wicked carried us away in captivity.' If you're not familiar with this song by Boney M, then ask your parents (or grandparents!) or look it up online.

The people of Judah are in exile in Babylon, feeling very sorry for themselves. But prophets, such as Isaiah, spoke about God bringing the people back to Judah but also having a bigger and better restoration plan in mind.

Today's reading talks about a servant 'pierced for our transgressions... the punishment that brought us peace was on him' (Isa. 53:5). The book of Isaiah was written 600 years before Jesus was born but contains many detailed prophecies about Him. God had not forgotten His people – He had a plan. Not only will Jesus come to save the Jews but everyone 'to the end of the earth' (Isa. 52:10).

God's plan to reign in and through the people of Israel had been thwarted by sin and then exile. Although some of the Jews would return to Judah, things were still not ideal. It is only with the arrival of Jesus that the problem with sin would be dealt with completely. Through His death and resurrection, Jesus would save Israel *and* the world.

CORE THEME | THE BIBLE 2

❝ ## *Share*

'My favourite Bible character is Paul because he remained faithful to God even though he was imprisoned, beaten and shipwrecked.' (Ethan, 17)

A light in the darkness

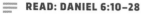

READ: DANIEL 6:10–28

KEY VERSE V26
'I issue a decree that in every part of my kingdom people must fear and reverence the God of Daniel. "For he is the living God and he endures forever."'

Last November, iconic buildings such as the Houses of Parliament, Marble Arch, and the Colosseum were flood-lit red as part of Red Wednesday to raise awareness of the fact that today, as in Old Testament times, people suffer persecution because of their faith.

Daniel was one of a number of highly talented people exiled to Babylon. Despite being in a strange land, Daniel and his friends remained true to God. This story must be an encouragement to all people who are suffering persecution for their faith. It does not mean that God will always rescue us from any harm in such a dramatic way but it does reassure us that, ultimately, all will be well if we commit ourselves to God. In this story, one man's light shone; since then millions of people have continued to shine God's light to the world.

Following Jesus sometimes means that life will be hard. This is particularly true in some parts of the world where Christians live in hostile environments. Could you get involved in this year's Red Wednesday on 27 November? Maybe you could organise a cake sale or simply wear something red to show your support. Visit acnuk.org for more information.

CORE THEME | THE BIBLE 2

❝ *Share*

'My favourite Bible verse is John 3:16, "For God so loved the world that he gave his one and only Son, that whoever believes in him shall not perish but have eternal life."' (Cam, 15)

It's time!

≡ **READ: LUKE 2:1–20**

KEY VERSE V11
'Today in the town of David a Saviour has been born to you; he is the Messiah, the Lord.'

CORE THEME | THE BIBLE 2

→ Some of the Old Testament prophecies are now being dramatically fulfilled in Luke's Gospel. God has been busy planning events in advance so that Caesar's decree would result in Joseph and Mary travelling to Bethlehem, thus fulfilling Micah's prophecy regarding the birthplace of Jesus. God then placed a special star in the sky to guide the wise men to Bethlehem and worship this new king. Luke is keen that we get the point that Christ's coming had been planned and links back to the story of God's people in the Old Testament.

This tiny baby is part of God's plan and He 'will cause great joy for all people' (v10). Jesus was not randomly sent into the world but came at just the right time to enable people who trust Him to do what they were created to do: enter a relationship with Him. And that they would be a blessing to the whole world – just as God promised Abraham. The rule and reign of Jesus would not be the political solution to overthrow human oppressors as hoped for but would mean living a new kind of life following Him.

As far as we know, Jesus had a fairly normal childhood in a simple home, learning a trade from His father, until the time came when He would start His teaching ministry and turn the world upside down.

❝ *Share*

64

'My favourite Bible character is Job because he kept faith in God throughout his troubles.' (Daniel, 15)

#Jesus

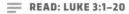

READ: LUKE 3:1–20

KEY VERSE V16
'John answered them all, "I baptise you with water. But one who is more powerful than I will come, the straps of whose sandals I am not worthy to untie. '

Last year, Selena Gomez had the most Instagram followers with 136 million followers, while Cristiano Ronaldo came second with 124 million followers. Bearing in mind that the total population of the UK is 53 million, these are huge figures!

We can safely say that John the Baptist did not have millions of followers but he did draw quite a crowd. He was a prophet calling people to repent and turn to God. At this point, the people of Israel were back in their homeland but under the power of the Romans. Although there were pious groups such as the Pharisees, the Israelites had largely turned their backs on God.

John's message was not just to 'try hard' but to return to the ways of God and have concern for the poor, honesty in taxation, fairness and contentment. John is known as 'the Baptist' because of his practice of baptising people, which was symbolic of making a new start. He had many followers, but he was very clear that it was Jesus who everyone should ultimately follow.

Are there ways you could subtly draw the attention of your friends and followers towards God? Maybe by posting a picture of a beautiful sunset or leaf? You never know, it might lead to some interesting discussions.

 Share

'The Bible reminds me that when I am going through struggles of daily life, God is still there.' (Marcus, 18)

CORE THEME | THE BIBLE 2

Life begins... again

READ: JOHN 3:1–21

KEY VERSE V16
'For God so loved the world that he gave his one and only Son, that whoever believes in him shall not perish but have eternal life.'

Today's reading describes a conversation between Jesus and a Pharisee called Nicodemus. The Pharisees were a strict religious sect who knew a lot about the Old Testament laws and history. So Jesus challenging Nicodemus would be like asking Brian Cox if he really understands physics.

The phrase that Nicodemus is failing to grasp is: 'no one can see the kingdom of God unless they are born again' (v3). This is understandable as it is quite a difficult concept for most people. The phrase 'born again' is only used in the New Testament and is best translated as 'born from above'. Through the Holy Spirit, God imparts a new kind of life that will stir us to live in the ways that Jesus taught. The Holy Spirit is someone who gives us a gentle nudge to do something or stop doing something. When we are born as babies, we start to live physically; when we are born from above, we start to live spiritually.

This conversation also includes one of the most quoted verses in the Bible: John 3:16. It sums up the whole message of the Bible – God really, really, really loves us. *Everyone* who puts their confidence in Jesus will enjoy a new kind of life now and for eternity.

66 *CORE THEME | THE BIBLE 2*

66 *Share*

'My favourite Bible character is Esther because she had the courage to speak out and save her people, despite the danger.' (Theo, 16)

Weekend

2/3 NOV

Shake off your doubts

READ: LUKE 4:14–29

KEY VERSE V18
*'The Spirit of the Lord is on me, because he
has anointed me to proclaim good news to
the poor.'*

'OK people hear the news, I got something
to yell about... Good news, Wakey wakey,
Good news, Shake your ass.' These are the
catchy lyrics from *Nativity!* Unfortunately,
the people of Nazareth weren't exactly
responding that way about homeboy, Jesus.
They were shaking their fists in horror that
this man who they had known from a young
age was claiming to liken himself to Elijah and
Elisha, their revered prophets.

Jesus had just returned from spending 40
days in the desert. He had totally trashed
Satan's attempts to tempt Him. He went
straight to the synagogue and announced that
He was ready to heal the blind and set the

oppressed free. Was there an orderly queue to take advantage of what Jesus was offering? Not quite. Instead of being delighted that someone wanted to help them, they were immediately suspicious and asked, 'Isn't this Joseph's son?' (v22). The atmosphere quickly turned really sour and they tried to kill Him.

Fortunately, there were many other places where people recognised Jesus as someone who spoke with authority and backed up His teaching with action. At the time, the poor were regarded as being beyond God's blessing, but Jesus challenged all that. The kingdom of God – God acting in the world – was being revealed in the miracles of Jesus. Something special was happening in Israel that had not been known and seen for hundreds of years. In the Gospels, there are 37 different recorded miracles... but very few take place in Nazareth.

 ### Think

Could doubt and suspicion be preventing you from accepting the good news about Jesus? Ask God to give you the faith to go for it and take advantage of what Jesus wants to do for you.

*Mirrorball Films, 2009

Learning by example

READ: LUKE 9:1–17

KEY VERSE V17
'They all ate and were satisfied, and the disciples picked up twelve basketfuls of broken pieces that were left over.'

Do you like cooking? Learning to cook is great if you have a recipe to follow but it is even better if you can watch someone else cooking. There are plenty of TV cookery shows on offer but not many that tell you how to feed a crowd of 5,000 people!

The account of the feeding of the 5,000 immediately affected more people than any other and signified Jesus' ability to do amazing things. All these people had followed Jesus to a remote place without bothering to pack a picnic first. There was no local supermarket to get some sandwiches and crisps. Can you imagine the faces of the disciples when they were told, 'You give them something to eat'? Jesus knew what was possible in the kingdom of God, of course, and wanted to stretch their thinking.

The disciples had just returned from going 'village to village, proclaiming the good news'. We don't know how long they had been gone or how successful their mission trips had been, but maybe Jesus wanted to see what they had learnt and how much their faith had grown. He listened to their suggestions but had a much better idea in mind: an extraordinary miracle. The disciples learnt that with Jesus extraordinary things *can* happen.

Share

'My favourite Bible verse is John 10:10: "I have come that they may have life, and have it to the full."' (Harriet, 16)

CORE THEME | THE BIBLE 2

A tale of two brothers

≡ **READ: LUKE 15:11–31**

KEY VERSE V32
'But we had to celebrate and be glad, because this brother of yours was dead and is alive again; he was lost and is found.'

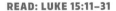

Requesting to have your inheritance before your parents had died would be shocking in New Testament culture. (It would be a bit odd now!) Even more shocking in the story, is the father who agrees to his son's request. After quickly squandering the money, the son decides to return home totally prepared to take on the role of a servant rather than a son. But his reception was not at all what he was expecting; his father was looking out for him, runs to meet him and welcomes him back with open arms.

There is another interesting character in this story: the older brother. He can't believe that his younger brother has been welcomed back, no questions asked. He, on the other hand, had faithfully remained, doing all the hard work but getting none of the credit. In a huff, he boycotts the family reunion party, preferring to stew on his own.

Jesus wanted His listeners to know that, like the father in the story, He has no problem welcoming back those who have made mistakes. The story doesn't tell us if the older brother changed his attitude, but let's celebrate when people want to have a close relationship with God.

There is a beautiful painting by Rembrandt called *The Return of the Prodigal Son*. Why not look it up online?

Share

'I like to read the Bible because it has helped me through stressful situations.' (Samuel, 16)

CORE THEME | THE BIBLE 2

Are you a remainer?

READ: JOHN 15:1–17

KEY VERSE 5

'I am the vine; you are the branches. If you remain in me and I in you, you will bear much fruit; apart from me you can do nothing.'

Today's reading takes place around the time of the Passover meal that Jesus has with His followers. It is one of the last times He has with all of them, so He is keen to pass on some final words.

Jesus is once again trying to open the disciples' eyes to the fact that He is the Christ prophesied about in the Old Testament. He does this by carefully choosing familiar imagery that they would be familiar with by referring to Himself as 'the true vine' (v1). This would have rang bells as, in Isaiah 5:7, it says, 'The vineyard of the LORD Almighty is the nation of Israel and the people of Judah are the vines he delighted in.' By using the term 'true', He is saying that He will bless all nations way more than the people of Israel.

Jesus also wants His disciples to know that the love God has for Jesus is equal to that which Jesus has for them and us. Thanks to this strong love and connection with Jesus, we can rely on God's resources to help us. When we want what God wants then situations can be transformed. Connectedness with God will not save us from troubles, which can come to followers of Christ just as they came to Jesus, but we will not be alone – the Holy Spirit will be with us.

CORE THEME | THE BIBLE 2

❝ *Share*

'My favourite Bible verse is Jeremiah 29:11 because it reminds me of God's promises of love and truth for me, especially if I am struggling with uncertainty or identity.' (Grace, 18)

The end?

READ: MATTHEW 27:32–54

KEY VERSE V50
*'And when Jesus had cried out again in a loud voice,
he gave up his spirit.'*

The death of Jesus is at the heart of the Christian faith and most people are familiar with the Easter story. It might even be so familiar that it is easy to become desensitised to the full horror of His suffering.

After being found guilty of blasphemy in a mock trial, Jesus was flogged, tortured, stripped of His clothes, mocked, spat at, a crown of thorns pushed on to His head, and He was beaten around the head with a big stick. He would have been covered with bruises, bleeding profusely, exhausted and dehydrated. In this terribly weak condition, He had to pick up a very heavy and large wooden cross and carry it through the streets of Jerusalem to Golgotha with people shouting abuse.

Even after being nailed and hung on the cross, people taunted Him by saying, 'He trusts in God, Let God rescue him now.' But God didn't rescue Him, and Jesus died. *Why didn't God save Him?* Jesus' death was planned from the moment He was born. He took on all our sin that prevented us from getting close to God. Our heavenly Father loved us so much that He made a way for us to be forgiven. Through Jesus, we can now have a relationship with God. Jesus' death was horrific, but it wasn't the end...

Share

'My favourite Bible character is Elijah because he is very relatable to lots of people who are affected by depression.'
(Josh, 16)

Doubts

READ: MATTHEW 28:1–20

KEY VERSE V6
'He is not here; he has risen, just as he said. Come and see the place where he lay.'

He's alive! Yes, Jesus is alive. He had tried to mentally prepare the disciples about His death and resurrection, but they clearly hadn't understood. The two Marys were shown by an angel to the place where Jesus' body had been. Twice the angel had to say, 'He has risen', before instructing them to tell the disciples to go to Galilee.

Once they were all gathered in Galilee, they had a little praise party and worshipped the fact that Jesus was more powerful then death. Jesus then told them to 'go and make disciples of all nations' (v19). This is referred to as 'The Great Commission'. It is our mission too, as followers of Jesus, to tell others about Him.

This mission might not be easy and many people will not believe in the good news about Jesus. The two Marys had to be told twice that Jesus was risen, and in Galilee, 'some doubted' (v17). If there were some who doubted even when Jesus was right in front of them, we can be forgiven for having doubts sometimes ourselves. It takes faith to believe that Jesus was who He says He was, but let's hold on to that promise that Jesus says that He will be with us 'to the very end of the age' (v20).

CORE THEME | THE BIBLE 2

Pray

Heavenly Father, sometimes it is hard to comprehend that You rose from the dead for me. Please help me to believe, and open my mind, my heart and my eyes to see the wonder of Your perfect love for me. Amen.

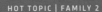
**WEEKEND
9/10 NOV**

FAMILY

What are you wearing?
READ: COLOSSIANS 3:12–17

KEY VERSE V14
*'Above all, clothe yourselves with love,
which binds us all together in perfect
harmony.' (NLT)*

Today's verses are quite a popular choice for readings
during a wedding service. They beautifully sum up
what a godly attitude towards our family actually
looks like in practice. Kindness, humility and patience
are all important qualities in making families work.
Above all, it's love that brings family members
together and keeps them together.

That might sound obvious, but it's surprisingly easy
to forget, and surprisingly tricky to live out. Love isn't
just a warm, fuzzy feeling. Love is a choice to commit
ourselves deeply to other people, to support them
and to put their needs before our own. Of course,

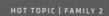

family life isn't always easy. Problems come, the people we live with sometimes do stupid things, and sticking with them can be difficult. When hard times come, the basic principle is: choose to love your family. It means being patient, kind, humble and forgiving. That's why we're encouraged to 'clothe ourselves' – it implies a deliberate action. Think about it – you make a choice as to what you wear each day. Even when it's the last thing on earth we feel like doing, we can 'clothe ourselves with love'. Realistically, we can only do this with God's help. He is the limitless source of love, and isn't ever going to run out of it!

In this second section on the subject of family, we'll concentrate on what happens when things go wrong within our families, with examples from the Bible to boot. We'll think about how we should respond and what it means to show love to our families during hard times.

Pray

Lord Jesus, thank You for showing us the perfect example of love. Please help me to love my family, whatever happens. And please help me to understand more about what real love means. Amen.

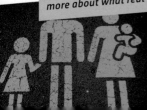

Rock bottom?

READ: GENESIS 37:18–36

KEY VERSES VV23–24
'So when Joseph came to his brothers, they stripped him of his robe... and they took him and threw him into the cistern.'

HOT TOPIC | FAMILY 2

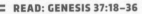

However you feel about your own family situation, there's no denying the truth about the state of Joseph's: it was pretty dysfunctional. Where to begin? There was favouritism, pride, deceit, anger, rivalry... (and very nearly murder). We mentioned at the weekend how important love is in keeping a family together, but in this family there doesn't seem to be much love around. This is a dark episode in Genesis, but it isn't the end of the story. God turns the whole situation around, as we'll see tomorrow, and uses some awful circumstances for the purposes of His kingdom. In the meantime, He hasn't given up on arrogant Joseph or his thoroughly unpleasant brothers.

God hasn't given up on you, either. If your family has a few problems, don't think that nobody understands what you're going through. God's seen it all before! Jesus Himself was misunderstood by the people closest to Him (eg Luke 2:41–50). And don't think that God couldn't possibly be interested in you. He achieved something incredible through Joseph's family and He can do amazing things in your family, too.

🔼 *Pray*
Commit your family into God's hands. Ask for His help in any difficult situations you're facing and ask Him to forgive you for anything you've done to make the situation worse.

Working things out

READ: GENESIS 45:1–15

KEY VERSE V5
*'do not be angry with yourselves for selling me here,
because it was to save lives that God sent me ahead
of you.'*

Yesterday, we saw Joseph in a horrendous situation. His
relationships with his brothers had broken down so badly
that they were ready to kill him. Eventually, they settled
for selling him as a slave. But now, years later, Joseph is
reunited with his brothers and is somehow able to forgive
them for what they did to him. How is that possible? As
Joseph looked back, he could see that God had been at
work in his life. Despite being abandoned by his brothers,
imprisoned and forgotten, he could see that God had a
plan. Through Joseph, God had saved Egypt from a famine,
and saved the lives of Joseph's family – and God had
developed Joseph's character and made him stronger,
wiser and more mature.

God wastes nothing. He can bring good from our most
painful experiences. It isn't easy to forgive our family
when they've said or done something that really hurt us.
But if we keep our eyes on God and begin to see His plan in
it all, forgiveness is possible. We can be reconciled to our
family and move on.

 Think

*Do you need to forgive anyone in your family for anything?
Has God brought something good out of your painful
experiences for you or other people?*

*Remember, forgiving someone is not the same as saying what they did was OK.
If you're affected by the issue of abuse, talk about it to an adult you trust.

HOT TOPIC | FAMILY 2

Even in hard times

READ: JOHN 19:16–27

KEY VERSE V26
'When Jesus saw his mother there, and the disciple whom he loved standing nearby, he said to her, "Woman, here is your son"'

Even in His most crushing and agonisingly painful moments, Jesus still cared about those closest to Him. He knew that His death would leave His mother and His best friend grieving, and Mary possibly alone, so He brought the two of them together to care for and support each other. In His death, Jesus wanted to bring healing to those closest to Him, and as a result, John would then take Mary into his home and take care of her.

Through Jesus, there is still hope when our families disintegrate. After fierce arguments, after a divorce, even after someone dies, Jesus can heal our families, bring us closer together and give us hope for the future. So, if you're going through a tough family situation at the moment, or know someone who is, pray that God would use the challenges being faced to deepen and strengthen relationships. Family was always God's plan and He still cares about our families today. What's more, God can give us the strength to keep on loving our families when we feel like we're at the end of our tether. Even if loving your family seems impossible, God can give you the strength to persevere.

HOT TOPIC | FAMILY 2

➕ *Challenge*

Have you given up on a relationship within your family because it just seems hopeless? Pray for God's healing in this relationship. Be open to God prompting you in ways to help heal this relationship, too.

Love and loss

READ: JOHN 11:1–7,17–44

KEY VERSE V36
'See how he loved him!'

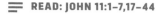

It's a terrible situation for a family to face: a sudden and untimely death. It's crushing. It seems so unfair.

Even when an elderly relative has lived a long, full and happy life, and has gone to be with Jesus, it can be really difficult to come to terms with their death. So, when we lose someone we love tragically young, it's even harder to get our heads around. Mary and Martha had just lost their brother, and what's more, they'd sent an urgent message to Jesus to come and heal him; but He didn't turn up until Lazarus was already dead. Their emotions must have been all over the shop. So what did Jesus do? Start with verse 35, but then read on!

This story doesn't give us answers as to why people close to us sometimes die, but it does give us a little insight into how Jesus feels about this whole thing. He grieves alongside us. He is close to us, wants to comfort us and let us cry and ask questions. And, above all, He gives us hope. He is the resurrection and the life. When someone close to us dies, Jesus might not bring them back to life but, whatever happens, He is right there with us to comfort us and give our families hope for the future. If you're grieving right now, or know someone who is, know that Jesus cares about you *so much*.

HOT TOPIC | FAMILY 2

 Pray
Thank Jesus for being with you, whatever happens, to understand, comfort you and give you hope.

Fear vs reality

 READ: GENESIS 33:1–11

KEY VERSE V4
'But Esau ran to meet Jacob and embraced him; he threw his arms around his neck and kissed him.'

Have you ever done something you know is wrong, got away with it, but lived in fear of being found out? Maybe as a kid you broke something, managed to cover it up, but were terrified of confessing to your parents in case they hit the roof and grounded you for the rest of your life. But when the truth finally did come out, their reaction was actually very gracious and forgiving. Have you ever experienced that kind of scenario?

In Jacob's case, he'd betrayed his brother in a major way. When Esau came looking for him, Jacob thought there was a real possibility that his life was in danger. As it turned out, Esau only wanted to forgive him and move on. When we've hurt a family member, we can tie ourselves in knots to avoid them or keep the secret, out of fear of how they'll react. But often our fear of their reaction is far worse than the reality. Let's keep talking. It makes it much easier to say sorry, be forgiven and move on. Try to keep the channels of communication as open as you can – especially with those in your family. It makes tackling those tricky situations, and areas of potential conflict, a lot easier.

 ## *Challenge*

Are you avoiding someone in your family? Are you keeping a secret because you're afraid of how the person will react? Have the courage to make the first move and say sorry.

Weekend

16/17 NOV

Sticking together

READ: RUTH 1:1–22

KEY VERSE V16
'Where you go I will go, and where you stay I will stay. Your people will be my people and your God my God.'

When hard times come to our families, our choices make a big difference. Our choices can bring our family members closer together, let relationships drift or even create a divide that wasn't there before. Ruth and Orpah both faced the same choice: to go their own way and try to make their own lives more comfortable, or to commit themselves completely to their mother-in-law and go with her. Orpah chose to go her own way, and we never hear any more about her. Ruth committed herself to Naomi, and some incredible blessings followed.

Ruth's first husband had died, as had her brother-in-law and her father-in-law. But

Naomi wasn't her only option – she could have gone back to her hometown and remarried. She might even have found herself someone rich and successful, and lived out the rest of her life comfortably without giving Naomi a second thought. But this woman knew where her loyalties should really lie, and stuck with the mother-in-law she had come to love and respect. At the time, she had no idea that this, the more difficult path, would end up being the road to a much happier happily-ever-after!

For us, the choices aren't always that stark. But when one of our relatives is suffering there is still a choice to make. Will we choose to act in a way that shows love and commitment? Or will we just let them get on with it by themselves? Even if it means sacrificing our own comfort, or being prepared to be inconvenienced for a while, it's important that we show up for those we love. Let's be committed to our families. Let's remember that our choices are important in this. God can bless and unite our families if we choose to show love and commitment.

 ## Think

Who in your family is struggling at the moment? How can you show love and commitment to that person?

Feet first

READ: JOHN 13:1–17

KEY VERSE V14
'Now that I, your Lord and Teacher, have washed your feet, you also should wash one another's feet.'

When you're asked to do something to help at home, what is your reaction? Do you get on and do it? Do you do it but moan about how unfair it is? Or do you think of as many excuses as possible for not doing it? Let's be honest – we've all moaned and complained when we've been asked to tidy our rooms or do the washing up and we're just not in the mood.

But Jesus really challenges this attitude. When He washed His disciples' feet, Jesus was putting Himself in the position of the lowest-ranked servant, washing the dirty feet of His friends (sandals didn't offer much protection against the dust, filth and animal dung on the roads they'd have walked along).

Jesus' actions communicated that He put other people before Himself. Jesus challenges us to do what He did and make a habit of serving other people. This includes our family. What might it look like if we were willing to put our family's needs before our own? It might not mean literally washing their feet, but it might mean washing the dishes. It might not mean laying on a huge feast, but it might mean cooking the dinner once in a while. Our attitude and our actions should put other people first. That includes the people we live with.

Challenge

How can you put Jesus' challenge into practice at home? What does 'washing your family's feet' mean for you?

HOT TOPIC | FAMILY 2

Let it go

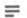

READ: MATTHEW 5:21–26

KEY VERSE V24
'First go and be reconciled to them; then come and offer your gift.'

The *San Francisco Chronicle* once reported on a man being sentenced to five months in prison for gunning down an ostrich. After a night of drinking, the man had trespassed onto an ostrich ranch with a few friends. One of the startled ostriches lashed out, kicking two of them to the ground. Enraged by this attack, the men hurried home, returning soon afterwards with a rifle and a shotgun to enact their revenge.

Anger is a dangerous thing. Anger and harsh words can lead to violence alarmingly quickly and easily. This may be why Jesus uses such strong words when He speaks against anger. Perhaps Jesus urges us to settle an argument quickly because He knows how things can escalate if we don't deal with our anger. Certainly, when we're angry, it spoils our relationships with people around us and with God. This is particularly important when we have to live with the person we're angry with! So let's clear the air quickly when we are angry with someone at home. Sometimes, it really is in our best interest to just let something go. Don't let an argument fester. Be prepared to give and receive forgiveness. And certainly sort out the problem before you come to worship God.

HOT TOPIC | FAMILY 2

Think

Is there anyone in your family who you need to settle an argument with? Ask God for His help to resolve things, and then make the first move to clear the air.

The power of forgiveness

READ: MATTHEW 18:21–35

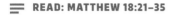

KEY VERSE V21
'Lord, how may times shall I forgive my brother or sister who sins against me?'

Forgiving someone when they've wronged you can be hard. And to keep forgiving that person over and over again is really hard. So why does it matter? First, for as long as we refuse to forgive that person, we're tying ourselves to the past and to our own anger and bitterness. So when we forgive someone, we don't just set them free from a grudge, we set ourselves free, too.[*]

Second, as Jesus points out in this parable, when we forgive a person, we're following God's example. God has forgiven us for everything we've ever done wrong, so in comparison it's a small matter for us to forgive each other.

Finally, if we're holding on to a grudge, we're holding back a part of our lives from God. This gives the devil a chance to hold us back in our relationship with God. There's no denying that forgiveness can be hard, but choosing to forgive someone is godly, healthy and liberating. And when we live with the person we're angry with, forgiving that person and healing our relationship with them is particularly important.

✚ Challenge
Is there someone you need to forgive – even if they haven't apologised? Ask the Holy Spirit to help you.

*Forgiving someone doesn't mean saying that what they did was OK. If someone has been seriously bullying or abusing you, get help. Talk to an adult you trust or contact ChildLine.

HOT TOPIC | FAMILY 2

Truth talking

READ: PROVERBS 24:23–26

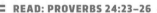

KEY VERSE V26
'An honest answer is like a kiss of friendship.' (NLT)

HOT TOPIC | FAMILY 2

It's likely that we've all done it: saying 'Oh, it's fine' to get out of a confrontational situation. We don't want to upset the apple cart, so even if someone has asked us what the problem is, we squirm out of the conversation just because we don't want to risk being a little bit uncomfortable. But honesty, the Bible tells us, really is the best policy – as long as we remember that whatever we say, we need to treat people with kindness and respect. But even tough truths need to come out. If we allow problems in our relationships to go unaddressed, it usually ends up in further upset, resentment, or drifting apart.

Of course, when tackling these difficult conversations, we need to be sensitive (Eph. 4:15), but, sometimes, it's only by speaking the truth that we can address a problem. It's not easy to tell someone something they don't want to hear, but they'll often respect us more for our honesty. And it works both ways! Even if it's a bit awkward at first, how much would you appreciate someone you love gently explaining to you how your actions/habits/attitude makes them feel? Allow your pride to take that initial hit, and then thank them for their feedback. It's a beautiful thing!

Pray
*Lord Jesus, please help me to be honest with my family,
to love and respect them and tell them the truth. Amen.*

All about love

READ: 1 CORINTHIANS 13:1–13

KEY VERSE V7
'[Love] always protects, always trusts, always hopes,
always perseveres.'

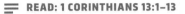

So we end this section of readings as we started it. It all
comes back to love. I wonder how well you display the
characteristics of love spoken about in this passage. Read
verses 4–7 again and try substituting your own name
for 'Love' and 'It'. Can you really say that you are patient,
kind, not rude or irritable and all the rest? The idea of this
isn't to make you feel bad about all your shortcomings,
but it's quite a challenge, isn't it? Now swap your name
for 'God'. Now it works! That's the God who has you, and
your family, safe in His hands. When you're struggling to
choose to love them, ask God for an extra dose. We can't
do this all on our own.

Perhaps you belong to a really tight-knit family, where
you're all really close and swift to sort out arguments. If
that's you, then that's great – keep God at the centre of
things, and carry on praying for each other. But if things
aren't so great with your family relationships, or you've
been through some really tough times together, ask God to
do something amazing. With His help, and with a resolve
to keep loving each other, we can overcome. He can work
all things for good (Rom. 8:28). Let's choose to love our
families, no matter what.

HOT TOPIC | FAMILY 2

 ## *Think*

*What have you learned through these readings on Family?
How will your attitude to your family change because of this?*

CELEBRATE

Party time
READ: LUKE 15:1–10

KEY VERSE V10
'there is rejoicing in the presence of the angels of God over one sinner who repents.'

As we come to the second half of our look at celebrating, there's some fantastic news waiting to blow your mind. You may remember that we learnt that God wants you to celebrate Him – not just by smiling a little when you think of Him, but *really* celebrating Him. Well, get this: God celebrates you! Not only does He love you (which you may have heard so many times that it's lost all impact), but He celebrates you.

In today's reading, Jesus tells these two parables, the lost sheep and the lost coin, mainly in response to the Pharisees' complaint about what He was doing.

Jesus had been eating dinner, but it was who His company was that caused the problem. Prostitutes and mafia bosses probably weren't high up on many people's guest lists, but there Jesus was, sitting and eating with them. In fact, He seemed to prefer their company to that of so-called 'good' people.

To explain His thinking, Jesus used everyday stories about sheep or coins being lost, the energy spent in searching for them, and then the great joy in finally finding them. 'Those insignificant people,' Jesus seems to say, 'who you don't think matter – well, they matter to me!' And He says that when one of these people turns to Him, the whole of heaven breaks out into party mode. That's right – whatever they're doing up there, it all gets thrown up in the air as they pull the party poppers and celebrate that one more person has been saved by Jesus!

Think

What do you think the parties in heaven look like? Is there dancing? What are they singing? Has there ever been one of those parties for you? If you have repented and turned to Jesus, then one of these was thrown in your honour! If you haven't, this might be the day to give the angels an excuse to get their groove on!

Welcome home!

READ: LUKE 15:11–25

KEY VERSE V24

'"this son of mine was dead and is alive again; he was lost and is found." So they began to celebrate.'

Yesterday, we read about the lost sheep and the lost coin. Today, we're looking at the lost son. It seems that Jesus really, really wanted those religious guys to get the point – or maybe they were just a bit slow. In either case, it apparently took Him three stories to get it across to them!

As we saw on 5 November, it's fascinating to see what the father in this story does when his son returns to him. It provides such an incredible portrayal of God the Father, and probably shocked Jesus' listeners. To have a man, who in those times would be seen as the head of the household, running to meet his son (v20) was unheard of in Jewish culture. It was seen as totally inappropriate, even humiliating. Yet, the father does this in celebration of his returning son.

Next, the father pulls out all the stops in putting on a party for his son. No expense is spared as he throws this spontaneous celebration of his son coming home. There are catwalk-ready clothes, the best food, music and dancing. This is an image of that party we learnt about yesterday – God pulls out all the stops in celebrating His returning children, when we decide to follow Him.

 Pray

Father, thank You for caring so much about me and for throwing a huge party for me. Use me to show other people who You are and what You're like. Amen.

What a tune

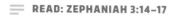

READ: ZEPHANIAH 3:14–17

KEY VERSE V17
'He will rejoice over you with joyful songs.' (NLT)

Most of us will have heard many times that God loves us. It's one of those Christian facts that's drilled into us. But, sometimes, we can forget what that love actually means and looks like. So here's one fantastic, intimate and meaningful image of what God's love for you looks like: He's singing songs about you. The good kind. In fact, the incredible kind – He's rejoicing.

This passage was originally written to show the relationship God had with the nation of Israel, His people, but it also reflects God's thoughts on His relationship with you, because you are one of His people! You may feel sometimes that you pray prayers and sing songs, and they go off into a big silence. This verse teaches us otherwise. Not only does God speak to you, through the Bible, through other people and directly to you in words and images but, somewhere in a heavenly dimension, He is also singing a song about you. We sing songs and He sings back.

If you ever feel like you're nothing special, remember that God is so excited about who you are that He quite literally bursts out in song over you. You cause Him to celebrate!

 ## *Challenge*

Find a quiet spot and make yourself comfortable. Talk to God about today and then ask Him to show you a bit of His song about you. If it helps, grab some paper or use your phone to write down anything that comes to mind.

HOT TOPIC | CELEBRATE 2

Thinking of you

READ: PHILIPPIANS 1:3–6

KEY VERSE V3
'I thank my God every time I remember you.'

So, God celebrates us. This teaches us something important, which is that we are worthy to be celebrated. And it also means that the people around you are worthy to be celebrated.

The letter to the Philippians is an amazing book of the Bible (why not read the whole thing sometime). If you had to give the book a theme, it would definitely be joy. This is extraordinary, because the author, Paul, wrote it in prison! But, time and time again in this letter he returns to the subject of joy – how much he has despite his circumstances, and how his readers should rejoice in God whatever happens.

Paul also says to the Philippians that every single time he thinks about them, he thanks God for them. And these are not muttered prayers, only said because he feels he has to. These are prayers filled with joy. Part of this joy comes from the Philippians continuing the work that he started, but he is also excited about what God is doing in them: the good work that has begun (v6).

Paul has understood that people are worth celebrating. God is doing great things in the lives of the people around us. Let's open our eyes to it!

 ## *Think*

Think about some of the great qualities that a few of your friends and family have, and celebrate these people before God. You might also want to send an encouraging text, email or card to one or two of them.

Dinner time

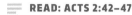

READ: ACTS 2:42–47

KEY VERSE V46
'They… met in homes for the Lord's Supper, and shared their meals with great joy and generosity' (NLT)

Today, we're taking a look at how the first Church celebrated together. While some people might think that the two words 'Church' and 'celebrate' don't belong in the same sentence, the first Christians show us that celebrating was at the heart of Church life.

Notice how this group of people seemed to be having a great time and enjoying each other's company. They regularly met up and had dinner together – and they loved it! They didn't care about stuff like how rich they were, in fact they sold their possessions and gave the money to the poor. Isn't it great that the description of the newborn Church focuses as much on practical things as on 'religious' things? Sure, they were praying and listening to teaching (v42), but they also saw sharing what they had as a huge priority. All done with joy. Church was the community that they did life with, and joyful celebration was as massive part of that.

And look what happened: more and more people became followers of Jesus. People looking on from the outside saw what the Church was like and wanted to be a part of it.

Think

In what ways does the description of the Early Church sound like your church or youth group? In what ways does it not? What could your church/youth group learn from these verses? Perhaps you could talk to your youth leader or church leader about some ideas you have.

HOT TOPIC | CELEBRATE 2

The after party

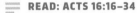

READ: ACTS 16:16–34

KEY VERSE V34
'He... set a meal before them, and he and his entire household rejoiced because they all believed in God.' (NLT)

Have you ever been to a baptism? Can you remember what it was like?

The Early Church baptised people as soon as they became Christians, not a few months later, not even a day later. In this story, we meet some of Paul's friends in Philippi who had just become new believers in the Philippian church (the people who received the letter we read from on Wednesday). Paul and Silas had got into trouble for doing good in the name of Jesus and were thrown into jail. Notice their celebration and praise of God under pressure – they were in the inner cell, feet in stocks, and there they were singing worship songs!

The jailer saw the work of God in releasing Paul and Silas from their bonds and he was desperate to be saved. It wasn't just him that was saved in the end, his whole family turned to Jesus. Without any delay, they were all baptised, then returned to the jailer's house to celebrate and bask in the joy of this amazing occasion with a dinner party.

Next time you're at a baptism party, make sure you really take in and celebrate how exciting it is that the person has turned to Jesus and publicly shown this.

➕ *Challenge*

Have you been baptised? The Bible says that being baptised shows the rest of the world that we follow Jesus. If you think you would like to do this, have a chat with your church leader or youth leader.

HOT TOPIC | CELEBRATE 2

Weekend

30 NOV/1 DEC

The real meal

READ: 1 CORINTHIANS 11:17–34

KEY VERSE V33
'So, my dear brothers and sisters, when you gather for the Lord's Supper, wait for each other.' (NLT)

What does taking Communion look like in your church? In some churches, you kneel at a rail. In others, you go up to the front. And in some, you are handed it by the person next to you.

Celebrating the Lord's Supper was part of the Church's identity pretty much from day one. It is mentioned in Acts 2 in the short description of the first Church, but was quite different then from what it is in most churches today. The Lord's Supper was a meal. A meal where the believers came together to share bread and wine to remember Jesus. It was a time of celebration.

In our passage today, the Christians in Corinth were being told off by Paul. Something in their sharing of this meal was going wrong. The problem was in how they were treating each other – they were divided, and some of them had become a bit selfish. They would rush ahead, eating and drinking all they liked, not caring that others were being left hungry (v21). That just wasn't the way that the Lord's Supper was meant to be, so Paul called them out on it. He told them they needed to remember what it was really about.

In our churches, many of us are so used to Communion that we gloss over what an amazing thing the Lord's Supper actually celebrates. It is supposed to remind us of our salvation – that Jesus went to the cross and died for us so that we could be totally forgiven. Romans 8:1 tells us, 'there is no condemnation for those who belong to Christ Jesus' (NLT). That is truly something to be thankful for!

✚ Challenge

Next time you take Communion, remember what you're really celebrating. Take a few moments beforehand to think about what Jesus did for you, and eat and drink with real thankfulness.

On the guest list

READ: LUKE 14:12–14

KEY VERSE V14
'God will reward you for inviting those who could not repay you.' (NLT)

Here we get some party-planning advice straight from the mouth of Jesus! We might be able to read into this passage some other 'more spiritual' meaning if we try but, at the end of the day, it's practical advice and shows us Jesus' love for the people who others might not care to include.

When people organise parties, there's usually a guest list in some shape or form. It's then that some people get quite flexible when thinking about who their 'friends' are, in order to include those they don't really know but whose presence at their party will make them look cool. Others may invite people who are really popular or rich, hoping that this will get them into that group of friends.

This is our human, selfish way of behaving. Jesus wasn't selfish when He was on earth. He loved the people who others didn't. He's not a fan of our way of manipulating people to get what we want. He tells us to invite those nobody else would invite, those whose presence won't raise our status. It's these people who may really need a friend. And these were the people on Jesus' guest list, so let's take some party-planning inspiration from Him.

Pray
Lord, show me who You want me to invite into my life, and give me wisdom for how to involve them in my social scene. Help me to not always consider myself first when choosing friends. Amen.

Feast your eyes on this

READ: LUKE 14:15–24

KEY VERSE V16
'A man prepared a great feast and sent out many invitations.' (NLT)

Jesus continues to teach about parties, but in this parable there is a definite second layer of meaning. Jesus is referring to the people of Israel as the original guests to the feast. When Jesus invited them to follow Him, lots of the Jewish people were far too busy with their own concerns to even seriously consider the invite. So, instead, He says that He will invite the people who are humble, and next, those who are from further afield – the non-Jews (most of us!).

But there are other important learning points here for us too. First, what Jesus invites us to, when He calls us to follow Him, is a party! If we let Jesus have His way, our lives, though challenging at times, will become an incredible adventure – a real celebration – as we trust God to guide us with the individual plans He has made for our lives. Second, there is a warning not to become too busy with life to hear Jesus' invitation to follow Him. Let's not let things like relationships, belongings or other commitments on our time take the place of Jesus. If we do, we are the ones who miss out.

Think

Fold a piece of paper in half. On one half, write a list of things that are important to you in life. On the second half, write down the things you spend most of your time doing. How do the two lists measure up? Do you need to change your priorities?

Can't stop the party

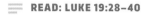

READ: LUKE 19:28–40

KEY VERSE V40

"'I tell you," he replied, "if they keep quiet, the stones will cry out.'"

The celebration of who Jesus is would happen whatever! That is what Jesus tells the Pharisees in this passage. They were upset because the crowds of people were praising Him as the Messiah. The very act of Jesus riding into Jerusalem on a young donkey was the fulfilment of the prophecy given in Zechariah 9:9. This was a big statement and the Pharisees didn't like it at all. They wanted Jesus to stop the crowds praising Him and simmer down. But Jesus explained to them that it wasn't as easy as that. If the crowds stop praising, the stones would start instead!

Then, just a few days later, the praise-filled cheers of the crowd changed into a demand to crucify Jesus. He who had looked like the triumphant Messiah was put to death on a cross. It seemed like the 'Jesus problem' was now done and dusted with – He was dead and surely the hype around Him would fizzle out too. But the story didn't end there, not at all: Jesus spectacularly rose from the dead. People all around the world are still praising Him to this day. Nothing and no one can ever stop the celebration of who Jesus is and what He has done.

 Pray

Jesus, along with the whole of creation, I celebrate You today. I give my praise to You and know that nothing can ever stop You being worshipped. Let all I do, say and think be glorifying to You today. Amen.

Wedding bells

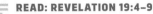

READ: REVELATION 19:4–9

KEY VERSE V7
'Let us be glad... For the time has come for the wedding feast of the Lamb, and his bride has prepared herself.'
(NLT)

Here's a dramatic passage if ever there was one. If anyone ever tells you that they fully understand the book of Revelation, they're probably lying! By its nature it's incredibly poetic and symbolic. But in this passage there are a few facts that are inescapable.

First, there will be some incredibly extravagant praise going on in heaven. There are crowds shouting out and falling down, the atmosphere is roaring and thunderous. Probably not your average Sunday morning!

Second, the celebration centres on something in particular. It's a party for the wedding between the Lamb and His bride. Now, this is when all the description starts to sound a bit weird. A Lamb marrying a woman? What?

This is, like much of Revelation, a piece of imagery. The Lamb, Jesus Christ, who was sacrificed to take away our sin (like a sacrificial lamb in the Old Testament), will finally be reunited with His beautiful bride, the Church. The Church goes through ups and downs, but the message here is that one day, the Church as a whole will be united with Jesus and will join in with His never-ending party.

 Challenge
Are there any ways that you could get involved in helping your church to worship Jesus right now? It might be helping out with a children's group, serving teas and coffees, or getting involved in the worship band. Talk to your youth leader.

HOT TOPIC | CELEBRATE 2

All together now!

READ: PSALM 150:1–6

KEY VERSE V6
'Let everything that has breath praise the LORD!'

We've come to the end of our study on celebrating. By now we've learnt a lot: celebrations were God's idea, He called Israel to celebrate Him, and He actually celebrates us! Yet, the most important thing to remember is that God deserves all the celebration you can muster. He gave you life and He saved you. He loves you and wants to be near you. There are so many things to celebrate Him for.

Our passage today is the very last psalm in the book of Psalms. It kind of sums up what they are all about – glorifying God. The writer of this psalm thought of loads of different ways in which God can be celebrated: dancing, singing and playing all sorts of instruments. Then he added, 'Let everything that has breath praise the LORD!' (v6). Birds, bears, mice, lions, poodles and giraffes – let them celebrate God! Let every single human being praise Him!

Philippians 2:10 says that every knee in heaven and on earth will one day bow before Jesus. If you only remember one thing from this study, remember this: God, above everything and everyone else, is worth celebrating.

Pray

Father God, I give You all the praise right now and celebrate who You are and what You've done for me. Please show me how to worship You in every area of my life, never forgetting how incredible You are. You deserve to be celebrated! Amen.

HOT TOPIC | CELEBRATE 2

**WEEKEND
7/8 DEC**

INTEGRITY

Basics for living
READ: JEREMIAH 22:1–5

KEY VERSE V3
'This is what the LORD says: do what is just and right'

In our previous look at integrity, we focused on our morals and ethics (including our conscience) and how these shape our lives. For the next two weeks, we are going to be looking at how we live with integrity, and considering some of the ethical decisions that affect us each day.

The Bible is full of commands God has given to His people. Some, like the Ten Commandments, we might know reasonably well. Other lesser-known commands, such as what to do if you get mould on your leather belt, might not be so familiar! (If you are curious about what to do in this scenario, turn to Lev. 13:47–49!)

God gave these commands to show us how to live – not to dampen our spirits. When we read the prophetic book of Jeremiah, we learn about God instructing His people to return to Him and His way of living. The people had turned their backs on God and weren't living the right way. Instead, they were worshipping false idols and not being fair to each other. God wanted them to do what was right, to live a moral lifestyle and treat others fairly and justly.

Although there are numerous commandments in the Bible, not every specific decision and choice has been covered. You won't find direct revelation about which college to go to and what subjects to take. You won't find revision techniques or the answers to your exams. However, God has enabled us to use our minds and has given us a set of instructions telling us to do what is just and right. Bearing these in mind will help us to follow God's commands in every situation and decision we make.

Pray

Ask God to speak to you over the next two weeks about how you can live in a just and right way. Ask Him to show you if you are not being fair to someone else and for the strength to put that right.

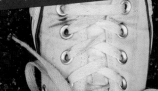

For richer, for poorer

READ: DEUTERONOMY 6:4–9

KEY VERSE V5
'Love the LORD your God with all your heart and with all your soul and with all your strength.'

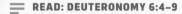

Have you ever been to a wedding ceremony for a relative or friend? Wedding services are usually wonderful occasions. As part of the service, the couple make vows to each other in front of all their friends, family and God. What is promised in the vows is no small thing. The bride and groom promise to love each other through sickness and health, for better and worse, and for richer and poorer. They also promise to give everything to each other and share everything: the last bit of pizza, their favourite ice cream, the TV remote and even do their share of the household chores!

This is what God wants from us: everything. He wants us to love Him with everything we have because He loves us. He wants us to love Him when we're healthy and when we're ill, when life is great and when it's tough. To love Him more than we do our possessions, securities and the people who love us. It's no small thing. We can start by wanting to follow His way rather than going our own. When we love God, we want to give everything to Him and follow what He says is right for us. Then God can really bless us by showing us the best path to go.

➕ *Challenge*

What are you holding back from God? Are there any areas in your life that you don't want God to change? Try talking to God today and ask Him to help you to allow Him to be part of everything in your life.

HOT TOPIC | INTEGRITY 2

Everybody needs good neighbours

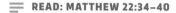

READ: MATTHEW 22:34–40

KEY VERSE V39
'A second is equally important: "Love your neighbour as yourself."' (NLT)

Have you ever watched the Australian sitcom, *Neighbours*? It was first broadcast in 1985 and is still going strong. *Neighbours* follows the lives of people living in the fictional setting of Ramsay Street. Well, these neighbours have had a rough time of it over the years. Storylines have included marital breakdown, teenage pregnancy, imprisonment, alcoholism, drug use, robbery, shootings and even murders. Two of the main families, the Robinsons and the Ramsays, have had a long history of rivalry. You might think twice before moving into this neighbourhood!

It's easy to love our neighbour when they're nice to us, but it's another thing when they don't like us. Our 'neighbour' is not just meant to be the people literally living next door, but those who we share this earth with. We're commanded to love the people around us – all people. It's one thing to love those who love us or are nice to us, but another to love those who are horrible to us.

How seriously do we take this commandment? It takes a strong person to take up this challenge and live it each day. But God knows that loving others is the best way for us.

Challenge

Who do you struggle to love? Think of a kind action or gesture to show love to someone you struggle to get on with and try to act on it before too long.

HOT TOPIC | INTEGRITY 2

It's so unfair!

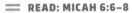

READ: MICAH 6:6–8

KEY VERSE V8
'No, O people, the LORD has told you what is good, and this is what he requires of you: to do what is right' (NLT)

What do you consider to be unfair? Perhaps it's buying a T-shirt only to discover it on sale the following week, or injuring yourself on the day of an important sports match. You may feel it unfair that your parents want you to be home early, or being a few marks away from a higher grade on a test.

Around the world, there are plenty of examples of social injustices in modern-day society. People are still treated unequally because of the colour of their skin. Low-income families are being referred to food banks in order to have something to eat. Elderly people are being neglected in certain care homes.

This passage challenges us to do what is right and to act in a just way instead of moaning about how we are being treated. Doing what is right can mean sticking up for those who are bullied, or not joining in with people who are breaking a window or scaring a neighbour. Doing what is right is an active command, not one that we sit around thinking about. It requires action. We need to be upholding justice, speaking out against what is wrong and acting on it. Seeking justice is a selfless act where we stop thinking of ourselves and start thinking about the needs of others.

Think

Think about the injustices you see in your area. What can you do to stop them? How can you motivate others to take action and help those who are suffering?

The power of forgiveness

READ: LUKE 23:26–43
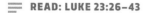

KEY VERSE V34
'Jesus said, "Father, forgive them, for they don't know what they are doing."' (NLT)

Has someone ever done something bad to you? Was it easy to forgive them? Probably not. We find it hard to forgive someone who has hurt us. The scars seem to stay with us. It makes it easier to forgive when the person tells us that they are sorry for what they have done. In many cases the relationship can be mended; we may begin to rebuild our trust in them again.

But what happens when they don't say sorry or seek forgiveness? Today's reading shows Jesus going through the most awful, painful experience and yet He asks the Father to forgive those who are responsible for this pain. The soldiers and the crowd don't say sorry or seek forgiveness from Jesus – yet He is ready to show mercy and to forgive.

If we hold on to the things done to us, resentment and bitterness can build up within us. It's like we keep ringing a bell of self-pity by talking about, and stewing on, a particular hurtful episode. Yes, we may have been treated badly but feelings of bitterness, given time, can cause us even more pain and suffering than the initial incident. We need to show mercy and forgive others – even when they don't deserve it. It's not the easy path to take – but it can make us stronger.

HOT TOPIC | INTEGRITY 2

Pray

Are there people you need to forgive? Pray, asking God to help you forgive them and to release you from resentment and bitterness. You may be surprised by how free this makes you feel!

Rules to live by

≡ **READ: MATTHEW 6:5–15**

KEY VERSE V10
'May your will be done on earth, as it is in heaven.'
(NLT)

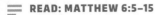

Have you seen the film, *Finding Nemo**? It is about a clownfish called Nemo. His father, Marlin, has told his son many times to stay close to the reef because Marlin knows all too well about the dangers that are out there in the wide ocean. But one day, curiosity gets the better of Nemo and he sneaks out from the reef towards a boat and is captured by a scuba diver.

Maybe you feel suffocated sometimes by rules and instructions from your parents and teachers. Do this; don't do that; be home by this time; don't wear that. Freedom to make your own rules might seem very appealing right now. But, yes, it's true: those looking after you usually know best. They want you to be healthy, safe and to make the most of opportunities. The same is true of our heavenly Father. His decisions are made with our best interests at heart. So it's even more fitting that we follow His will for us and do so humbly, knowing that His plans are better than our own as He knows what is best for us. To live God's way means to submit our own wishes to Him and follow His ways. It's as we say in the Lord's Prayer: 'Your will be done.'

🔾 *Think*

Reread Matthew 6:5–15 and pray the Lord's Prayer out loud. Consider the words you are saying. What would it look like if God's will truly was done in your life and in the world?

*Walt Disney Pictures, 2003

HOT TOPIC | INTEGRITY 2

Weekend

14/15 DEC

We are family

READ: JAMES 2:14–17

KEY VERSE V16

'you say, "Good-bye... stay warm and eat well" – but then you don't give... any food or clothing. What good does that do?' (NLT)

One incident in the life of Jesus is recorded three separate times in the Gospels of Matthew, Mark and Luke. While Jesus was teaching, He was told that His family were waiting outside. He replied 'Who is my mother? Who are my brothers?... Anyone who does God's will is my brother and sister and mother' (Mark 3:33–35). Now Jesus is not using the opportunity to be nasty or rude to His family; we know that family is important to Him. However, He was using the occasion to continue His teaching to the listeners about His spiritual family. We, of course, have people who we are related to by blood, but Jesus is talking about the strength of the ties we have with our spiritual family. The fact that we have been adopted into God's family means that those in our churches and in the worldwide Church are all part of our family.

Did you know that those around the world who do God's will are our Christian brothers and sisters? What a huge family we have! And so it's our duty to care for them as we would our own family. If we saw our own mother starving, would we feed her? Of course we would. We wouldn't want to see our family in pain or struggling – and yet we see it happening every day among our family living around the world.

Of course, it is good to be aware of *all* people, not just our Christian family, who are suffering around the world due to persecution, famine or war. What can we do? How can we help? Over the next week, we will be looking practically at our actions and how we can help all people across the world.

Challenge

Start thinking about what you can do to support others around the world. Why not try starting closer to home by doing odd jobs, cleaning cars or having a cake sale in order to raise funds for a charity?

Should I stay or should I go now?

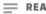

READ: ROMANS 15:25–29

KEY VERSE V26

'the believers in Macedonia and Achaia have eagerly taken up an offering for the poor among the believers in Jerusalem.' (NLT)

Every now and then, we hear on the news about a disaster or troubling situation somewhere in the world. On these occasions, as churches, it is right that we should pray, take up an offering and do what we can for the situation. The sad truth is that there will always be somewhere that needs our prayers and support. It's common to feel helpless and not know how best to help. Do we take up an offering like the believers in Macedonia and Achaia? Do we go and physically help like Paul? Or do we send others to go – like the church in Greece?

The important thing is to be willing to do something for God. The prophet Samuel, as a young boy, said to the Lord, 'Here I am' (see 1 Sam. 3). It's up to God what our response should be, whether it's to go or not. In order to know His will, we need to reply as Eli instructed Samuel to: 'Speak, Lᴏʀᴅ, your servant is listening' (1 Sam. 3:9). This may be through reading the Bible, through prayer or through other Christians.

If He says 'Go!' would you be prepared to leave it all and go? Or if He says 'Stay' would you be content with sending money and supporting those who go instead?

Pray

Tell God that you are here and willing to be used by Him. Spend some quality time in silence, reading the Bible or reflecting on what God may want you to do. Listen to what God has to say.

HOT TOPIC | INTEGRITY 2

Purchasing power

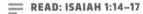

READ: ISAIAH 1:14–17

KEY VERSE V17
'Learn to do good. Seek justice. Help the oppressed. Defend the cause of orphans. Fight for the rights of widows.' (NLT)

Did you get a chocolate Advent calendar this year? You never get too old for those! Some Advent calendars contain chocolate from sustainably sourced fair trade co-operatives or cocoa farms that are 100% owned by farmers themselves. It's great to support Fair Trade suppliers, if you can. Look out for the Fair Trade logo on all sorts of food packaging as well as chocolate. Thankfully, choosing fair trade and ethical products has become much easier – whether it be bananas or clothes, an energy supplier or bank account. We can feel that we are doing our bit and making a difference, but there is always room for improvement.

God commanded His people through the prophet Isaiah to do good and seek justice. Using our money to buy goods that support the fair treatment of those who make the goods is important. But did you know that there are other ways we can voice our support of decent working conditions and a fairer deal for farmers? We can write to governments, asking for change. We can write to shops, commending them for the number of ethically-produced products they sell or requesting that they stock more. Or we can research the conditions of the workers and use the information to encourage others to support Fair Trade.

Think

What ways can you further seek justice for the oppressed? Where can you speak out against injustice?

HOT TOPIC | INTEGRITY 2

Speak up!

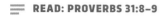

READ: PROVERBS 31:8–9

KEY VERSE V9
'Yes, speak up for the poor and helpless, and see that they get justice.' (NLT)

Those in marketing know that there is nothing like having a celebrity or a well-known vlogger endorse your product to help increase sales. YouTube videos and adverts on the television feature famous people singing the praises of a product, but do they actually regularly use that particular product? Do they use that shampoo or that type of broadband? Do they wear that perfume or shop in that supermarket? Are they being true to what they endorse? Or is it simply another job for them?

We might not become an influencer or appear in a TV advert endorsing a product. We might not have thousands of followers on our social media accounts – but we can reach our friends and families with news of justice for the poor.

The writer of Proverbs challenges us to speak up for those who are poor. This doesn't just mean buying fairly traded products but also endorsing them to those around us. It also means speaking about the difference buying these products might make and encouraging others to think about the wider world. Let's get radical and start the conversation!

 Challenge
Does your school or college sell ethically-produced goods in the cafeteria? Is this something you can promote or endorse? Perhaps you could suggest to your tutor having a fundraising day selling goods that contribute to a fair deal for the poor? It may even become a regular event!

HOT TOPIC | INTEGRITY 2

Root causes

READ: PROVERBS 21:2–3

KEY VERSE V3
'The LORD is more pleased when we do what is right and just than when we offer him sacrifices.' (NLT)

Have you ever watched Comic Relief, Sport Relief or Children in Need? They are great opportunities to raise awareness about a particular social need and anyone can get involved in the fundraising. Maybe you have done something yourself to raise money for a certain charity.

Comic Relief raised over £76 million in 2017, and Children in Need in 2018 raised over £50 million. These are fantastic amounts to support thousands of organisations and causes that help disadvantaged children and adults. Despite recession and economic difficulties, many people continue to give what they can, and incredibly, more and more money is raised each year.

You might wonder why there are still problems when so much money has been raised? Giving our money is commendable and it certainly helps to solve problems. But, maybe, we also need to ask the question: why are certain people in difficult situations in the first place? Are there long-term solutions that might address the root causes of poverty? How can our governments get involved and reach out to other countries in practical ways? Let's use our heads *and* our money to bring relief to those in need.

Think

Why is poverty still such a huge problem around the world? What are some of the root causes? Do a bit of research into this and see what ideas you can come up with that address the causes you find.

HOT TOPIC | INTEGRITY 2

Pass the love on

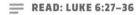 **READ: LUKE 6:27–36**

KEY VERSE V31
'Do to others as you would like them to do to you.' (NLT)

Christmas is a great time of year to show love to people. For example, we can send Christmas cards or e-cards to friends and relations. Even sending an encouraging text message can show how much we appreciate and love others. We love receiving these things ourselves, so it makes sense to pass the love on and do kind things for others, too.

The fact you are reading this means that you are better off than nearly a sixth of the population of the world who can't read. If you couldn't read, wouldn't you want someone to teach you? If you lived like over a third of the world without basic sanitation, wouldn't you want someone to help make it safe for you? If your child or younger sibling died because your family could not afford to immunise them, wouldn't you want immunisation for the rest of your family?

What we've learnt over the past few weeks and what we do about it can be summed up in today's verse. What are the ways in which you feel loved and how can you show other people in the world how much you love them?

 Pray

Lord, help me to treat others in the way I would want to be treated. Help me to show love and mercy to those who are suffering in our world and to play my part in bringing about a solution to the issues of poverty and injustice. Amen.

HOT TOPIC | INTEGRITY 2

THE BIBLE

Be prepared
READ: 1 PETER 3:13–18

KEY VERSE V15
'Always be prepared to give an answer to everyone who asks you to give the reason for the hope that you have.'

'You can point to the alleged miracles of the Bible... but they are nothing but old stories fabricated by man and then exaggerated over time." You may have heard other dismissive quotes and comments about the Bible such as that it is full of myths and contradictions. If we believe that the Bible is the Word of God, then these remarks might initially shock us and leave us grappling to find an appropriate response.

When negative opinions about the Bible come up in conversations, it's good to remember what our relationship is with that person and that they might not realise how they are offending us. It's also helpful to remember that we don't actually need to 'win' the argument or respond then and there. It might be better to wait for a more suitable moment to challenge their thinking. However, today's passage encourages us to 'always be prepared to give an answer.' So it's a good idea to have a response ready even if it is simply to say that you find the Bible helpful. Some of the common arguments against the Bible are:

- 'Science has disproved the Bible.' The Bible answers the important questions of 'who' and 'why' even if we don't fully understand the 'how'.
- 'The Bible is full of contradictions.' When asked to give an example, most people might struggle. Any differences in order of events affect very little of the text and there are no major doctrine contradictions.
- 'The Bible is too old to be believed.' The Gospels of Matthew, Mark, Luke and John include a lot of historical detail, which is backed up by archaeology.

Think

What are some of the objections to the Bible that you have heard? Why not jot them down and ask your minister or youth leader how they would respond.

*Dan Brown, The Lost Symbol (London: Bantam Press, 2009)

What an entrance!

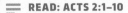

READ: ACTS 2:1–10

KEY VERSE V4
'*All of them were filled with the Holy Spirit and began to speak in other tongues as the Spirit enabled them.*'

According to Wycliffe, the complete Bible has been translated into 650 languages; the New Testament into 1,500 languages; and translation work is currently happening on 2,500 languages. You might think that is good progress but there are still many people globally who do not have a Bible in their own language.

After Jesus had returned to heaven, His followers were in Jerusalem at the same times as 'Jews from every nation under heaven' (2:5), all speaking different languages, were gathered to celebrate Passover (a bit like our Harvest Thanksgiving). Jesus' desire that His disciples would make followers of all nations is about to become true at a very opportune moment.

Jesus had promised a special helper for His followers who chose this moment to make quite an entrance. The Holy Spirit arrived in the form of a violent wind from heaven and tongues of fire. He also enabled the disciples to speak in different languages so the good news of Jesus could be heard by all people. The disciples needed the Holy Spirit's help before they could boldly take God's message worldwide. If they needed the Spirit to do this, we do too.

66 *Share*

'*My favourite Bible character is Joseph (Jesus' earthly father) because he is a remarkably courageous example of what it means to live sacrificially and be exactly where God wants you to be.*' (Grace, 18)

CORE THEME | THE BIBLE 3

I'm all shook up

READ: ACTS 10: 34–48

KEY VERSES VV34–35
'I now realise how true it is that God does not show favouritism but accepts from every nation the one who fears him and does what is right.'

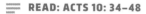

'I think there's just one kind of folks. Folks.' This is Scout's opinion in *To Kill a Mockingbird* by Harper Lee. Scout believes that each person is born equal regardless of their race, class or colour of skin. Unfortunately, other people in her town didn't share her view and were heavily prejudiced against certain groups of people.

Peter was similarly prejudiced against Gentiles (non-Jews). In the Old Testament, there were strict laws about who you could and couldn't eat with and what you could and couldn't eat. Despite being told to make disciples of all nations, it took a while for it to really sink in that God is willing to accept anyone who wants to know Him. God needed to intervene again in order for the Gentiles to hear the good news. He chose to use Peter who loved God but needed his thinking shaking up a little.

As Peter was preaching to Gentiles (non-Jews), the Holy Spirit fell on everyone just as it did at Pentecost. The speaking in tongues may not be a gift that a new believer receives, but the gift of the Spirit certainly is. This was crystal clear confirmation that God was intending to fulfil His promise to Abraham to bless *all* nations of the earth.

CORE THEME | THE BIBLE 3

66 *Share*

'I read my Bible when I am going through tough times and I need some inspiration.' (Marcus, 18)

All you need is love

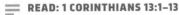

READ: 1 CORINTHIANS 13:1–13

KEY VERSE V13
'And now these three remain: faith, hope and love. But the greatest of these is love.'

Happy Christmas! Whatever you're up to today, may you know God's presence in an amazing way today as You celebrate His great love for you.

Today's reading – a great one for Christmas Day – is often read as a celebration of love at weddings. However, if we look at the previous chapter, we see that Paul was talking about love in the context of using spiritual gifts. A loving character is a fruit or a sign that the Spirit is in us. When we use spiritual gifts, we need to do so out of love. If we are using gifts such as speaking in tongues, prophecy, faith and giving in an unloving way then we are totally missing the point.

Some people place more significance on the more spectacular gifts but Paul says that even if he has amazing gifts such as speaking in tongues, without love he is nothing. We might feel that we have few spiritual gifts, if any, and we might be in awe of those who do. However, the most important spiritual gift is love and that is something we can all show to others.

➕ *Challenge*

In what ways can you show love to others this Christmas time? Maybe by taking some mince pies to a neighbour, or helping out with the washing up. Remember love is a spiritual gift too!

CORE THEME | THE BIBLE 3

Regal sons and daughters

READ: COLOSSIANS 3:1–17

KEY VERSE V17
'And whatever you do, whether in word or deed, do it all in the name of the Lord Jesus, giving thanks to God the Father through him.'

When Meghan Markle married Prince Harry and became the Duchess of Sussex, she chose to quit acting, close her website and shut down her social network accounts. These things aren't wrong, but she decided that they weren't helpful in light of her new role within the royal family.

At the beginning of today's reading, Paul reminds us that we 'have been raised with Christ' (v1). As Christians we are not the same as we were, we have a new outlook on life. We look forward to the day when Christ comes back but, in the meantime, there is work to be done. We are encouraged to share the good news of Jesus and be a blessing to others. In order to do this well, we need to let go of unhelpful habits and behaviours and replace them with positive virtues such as compassion, kindness and patience.

Meghan has Prince Harry to help her but we have our heavenly Father. We can let His Spirit dwell in us and guide us as to what to do. Everything we do matters to God, and, providing it is not sinful, it can be done 'in the name of the Lord Jesus' (v17). Wherever we are and whatever we are doing, let's remember our new status as children of the King and seek ways to serve Him.

CORE THEME | THE BIBLE 3

Share

'My favourite person to read about in the Bible is Jesus because He's the answer to everyone's problems.' (Harriet, 17)

Heroes of the faith

READ: HEBREWS 11:1–16

KEY VERSE V1
'Now faith is confidence in what we hope for and assurance about what we do not see.'

Stan Lee, who died last year, was a comic book writer and the creator of some of the extremely popular Marvel characters such as Spider-Man, Iron Man, Thor and Ant-Man. These fictional heroes use their superhuman strength to fight villains and avert disasters. Marvel films continue to attract huge cinema audiences with many films being released in recent years.

This reading in Hebrews is a list of people from the Old Testament who did things for God 'by faith'. Noah was warned about a flood and told to build an ark; Abraham was told to move to a foreign country and that he would be a leader of a great nation. They obeyed even though they weren't able to see, or fully understand, what was about to happen. By reading the Bible, we can see God's plan and purposes in retrospect. Looking back from the viewpoint of the New Testament we can see what God was doing all along. We have the whole Bible and can see God's faithfulness throughout time to all His people, but these heroes had far less to go on than us.

We can be heroes too, if we are open to hear God calling us to do things, by faith, for Him. Be assured that God is with you always, and that His plans for you may well blow your mind! What a great incentive to trust Him.

Share

'My favourite Bible verse is John 3:16 because it shows His love for me.' (Samuel, 17)

CORE THEME | THE BIBLE 3

Weekend

28/29 DEC

'greater worth than gold'

READ: 1 PETER 1:3–23

KEY VERSE V21

'Through him you believe in God, who raised him from the dead and glorified him, and so your faith and hope are in God.'

The World Watch List is Open Doors' annual ranking of the 50 countries where Christians face the most persecution. Persecution might take the form of being arrested for owning a Bible, not being allowed to meet to worship God, or not getting work or education because you are a Christian. This year, North Korea holds the number one spot, as it has for the last 18 years. There are between 50,000 and 70,000 Christians imprisoned in terrible labour camps in North Korea where they are worked like slaves and tortured; most are never able to escape. Christians are persecuted because they dare to believe in a higher authority than the ruling Kim family.

In today's reading, Peter was writing to people who were suffering persecution for their faith and he was keen to remind them why they needed to persevere. Jesus has given them a hope and 'an inheritance that can never perish, spoil or fade' (v4). In times of great trials, focusing on this will help their faith to grow and fill their hearts with joy for the future. Peter explained that God is fulfilling His promise to Abraham that all peoples in the world would be blessed through him. God's restoration of all things remains on track and Peter is encouraging persecuted believers by reminding them of this glorious truth.

It's unlikely that we will ever face the same persecution that our fellow brothers and sisters face in countries around the world. However, we may encounter ridicule, exclusion and scorn because of our faith in Jesus. When we do, we need to remind ourselves that we are God's special possession and continue to live as His holy people.

Pray

Loving Lord, please be with persecuted Christians around the world. In their darkest times, help them to remember that You are with them. Amen.

Walking in the light

READ: 1 JOHN 1:1–10; 2:1–6

KEY VERSE V9
'If we confess our sins, he is faithful and just and will forgive us our sins and purify us from all unrighteousness.'

Louis XIV reigned as king of France from 1643–1715. Also known as the Sun King, he believed that he was king by divine right and was not restricted by any written laws. In today's reading, however, John stresses that everyone has done wrong things, including kings, and if we think we haven't, 'we deceive ourselves' (v8).

Louis XIV may have likened himself to the sun but, in this passage, John describes God as light and 'in him there is no darkness at all' (1:5). When we walk with Him, we are walking in the light. Throughout his letter, John is concerned that his readers imitate God. Following Jesus' commands is a sure sign that God is at work within them. Living as Jesus did is not easy but this is John's challenge when he says, 'Whoever claims to be in him must walk as Jesus did' (2:6).

Becoming like Jesus might seem impossible and we can't do it in our own strength. We need God's Spirit to change us from the inside out so that we start to think, feel and act as Jesus would. John has experienced this during his time with Jesus and believed that others could too. This is a challenge for us to take on board today. Do we want to become more like Jesus? The Bible says we can.

Share
'I like to read the Bible in the mornings because it's an encouraging way to start the day.' (Theo, 16)

CORE THEME | THE BIBLE 3

The future's bright

READ: REVELATION 21:1–14,22–27

KEY VERSE V10
'And he carried me away in the Spirit to a mountain great and high, and showed me the Holy City, Jerusalem, coming down out of heaven from God.'

In heaven, will there be pearly gates? Will there be angels with golden halos? Will we have to wear white all the time? The answer to all these questions is: we don't really know. This reading from Revelation, however, gives us a small glimpse as to what heaven will be like.

We might not often think about it but one day, we will all die. As Christians we can be confident that when we die, we will go to heaven. God Himself, will come to dwell on earth and will renew all things. We won't have ghost-like bodies floating about somewhere but will enjoy renewed bodies in a new world that will have some similarity to what we are enjoying now.

The main difference between this earth and the new earth is that there will be no more death, crying or pain. His restoration plan will be complete and we will enjoy an eternal loving relationship with God.

As we look ahead to the coming year, we might worry about exams, our future and the future of our country. By giving us a glimpse of the future, God helps us to put things into perspective and, as we have seen in the Bible, we can trust that God is ultimately in control.

66 *Share*

'My favourite Bible verse is Jeremiah 29:11, "For I know the plans I have for you,' declares the Lord… plans to give you hope and a future."' (Theo, 16)

NOTES

ORDER FORM

4 EASY WAYS TO ORDER:

1. For credit/debit card payment, call 01252 784700 (Mon–Fri, 9.30am – 4.30pm)

2. Visit our online store at **cwr.org.uk/shop**

3. Send this form together with a cheque made payable to CWR to:
CWR, Waverley Abbey House, Waverley Lane, Farnham, Surrey GU9 8EP

4. Visit a Christian bookshop

YOUR DETAILS

Name:

CWR ID No. (if known):

Address:

Postcode:

Telephone No. (for queries):

Email:

SUBSCRIPTIONS (NON DIRECT DEBIT)	QTY	PRICE (INCLUDING P&P)			TOTAL
		UK	Europe	Elsewhere	
Mettle (1yr, 3 issues)		£14.75	£17.60	£18.75	
				TOTAL	

Please circle which four-month issue you would like your subscription to commence from:

Jan–Apr   **May–Aug**   **Sep–Dec**

Order direct from CWR or from your National Distributor. For a full list of our National Distributors and contact details, visit **cwr.org.uk/distributors**

Mettle is also available as a Digital Edition. For more information visit **mettleapp.org.uk**